YOUR PERFECT DIET MATCH

Diana Kelly Levey

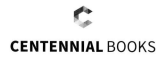

CENTENNIAL BOOKS

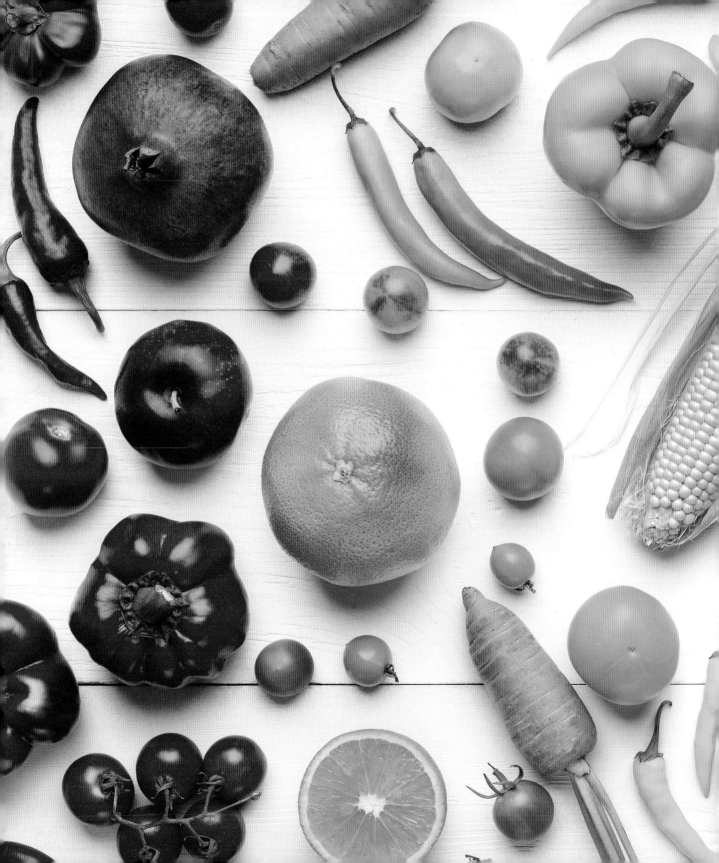

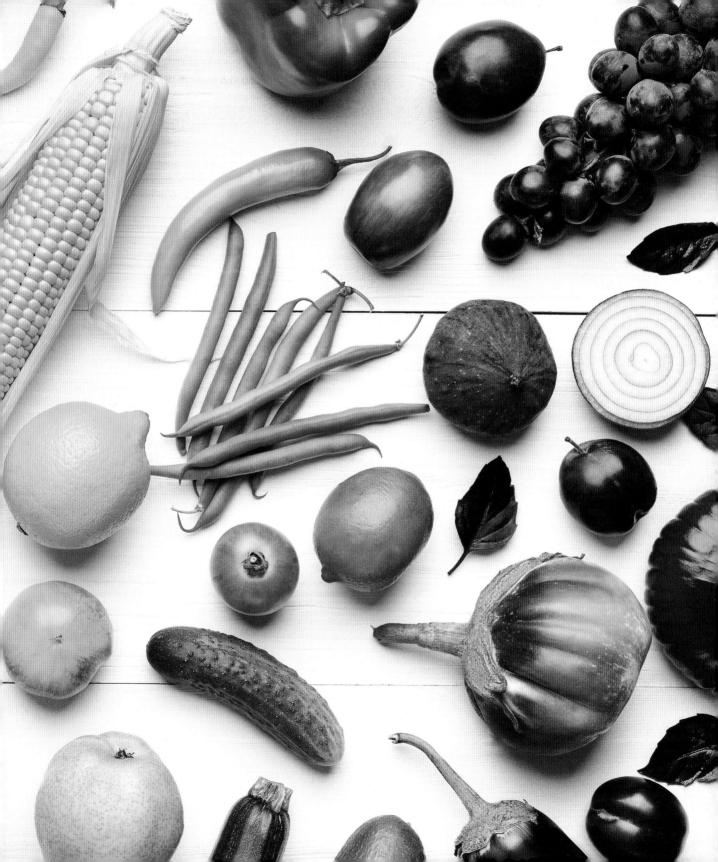

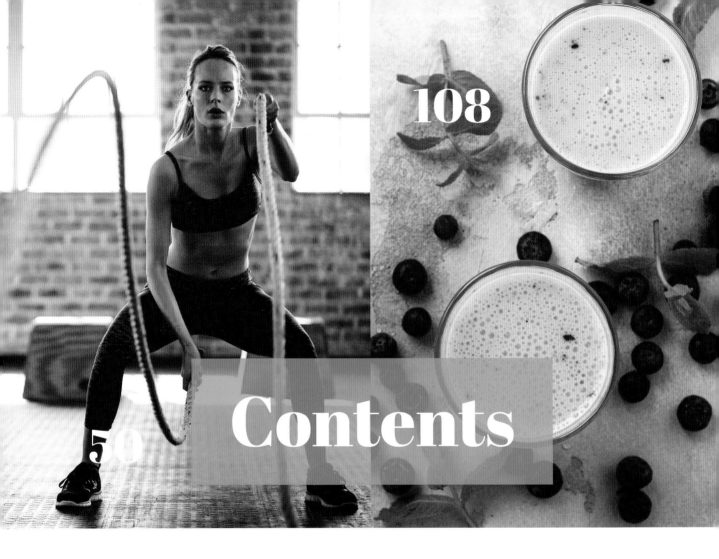

108

Contents

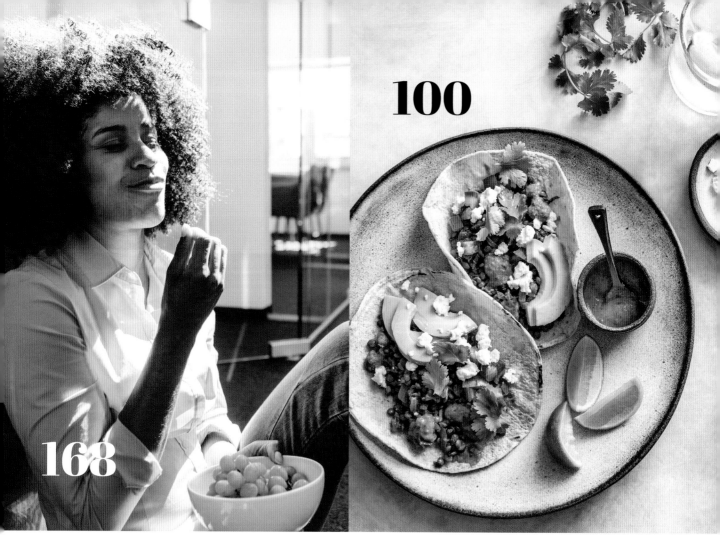

100

168

CHAPTER 3

LIVING WELL

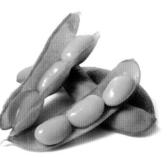

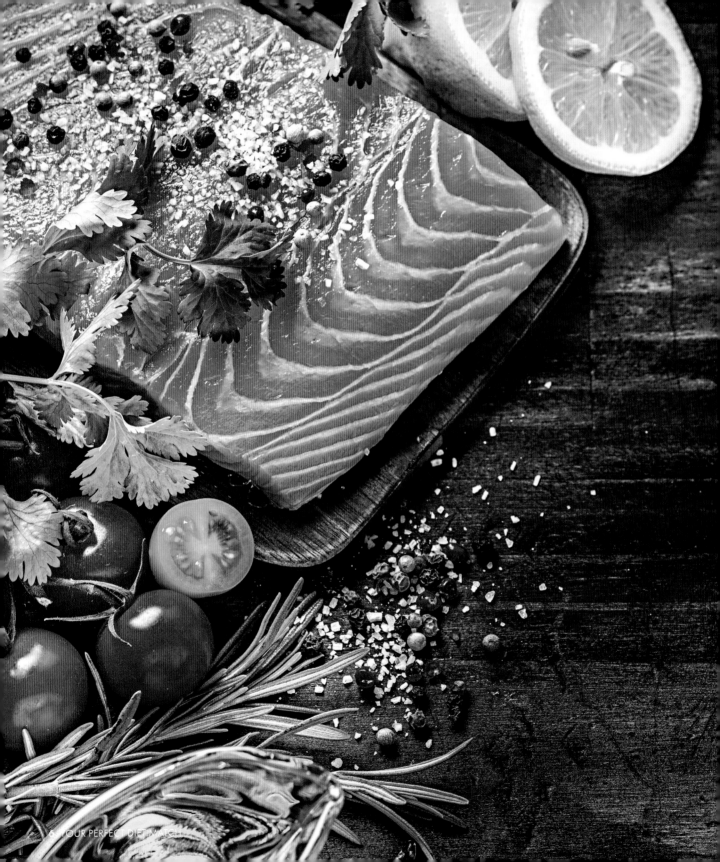

FIND YOUR MATCH

The key to weight-loss success is discovering a plan that suits your lifestyle.

Most dieters get off to a great start: You make shopping lists of healthy foods, then go home and chop, prep and cook three delicious meals and a snack a day. You're on your way, and the scale rewards your efforts! But then a week or two in, your boss moves a deadline up, your son announces he has a school project due tomorrow, and your car needs an urgent repair. Suddenly, your stress levels skyrocket, and all that shopping, slicing, dicing and vegetable-roasting takes a back seat. Meanwhile, you start craving forbidden foods, like chocolate, a burger or a glass of wine. Your initial enthusiasm and motivation are waning fast, and you're finding it tough to go the distance.

That's why it's so important to find a diet that's tailored to your lifestyle, personality, your food likes and dislikes, and your specific goals. After all, if one diet worked for everyone, there wouldn't be so many to choose from! Here are some factors to consider when selecting a plan:

You Can't Go a Day Without Bread, Meat or a Glass of Wine

If you love a good steak, a plant-based plan probably won't satisfy you. On the other hand, if you can't live without carbs, Atkins or keto may not be a good fit. And if you like real food, juicing is not for you. So before you pick a diet, think about what you really like to eat.

You Don't Have Time to Do Lots of Food Prep

If you hate grocery shopping and/or cooking, travel frequently or have a lot of time bandits in your life, you're better off with a diet that offers a lot of flexibility, as well as the ability to eat takeout or in restaurants (such as intuitive eating, Mediterranean or flexitarian) or offers shortcuts (frozen meals, like Atkins or WW).

You Just Want to Sit Down and Eat

If you're just here for the weight loss, not to do a lot of math problems, you'll want to avoid plans that involve weighing, computing calories or counting carbs. And if you don't want to do a lot of tracking and journaling, go for a plan that offers general guidelines, not strict rules, such as intuitive eating or The DASH, Lose Your Belly or Setpoint diets.

You Need to Drop Pounds Fast

While experts recommend losing no more than a pound or two a week, sometimes we need to slim down faster. Programs such as Atkins, Dr. Gundry's Diet Evolution, South Beach and The Dubrow Diet are organized in phases, which can help jump-start quick weight loss. People on low-carb diets often experience swifter initial slim-downs (although part of that is often water weight).

You Can't Deal With Starting Exercise and Dieting at the Same Time

You've decided you can swing the meal prep, but you just don't have time to start working out, too. You'll want to opt for a plan that doesn't require it, such as Atkins, keto or the alkaline diet.

You Want Champagne Results... But You're on a Beer Budget

Some diets—like Paleo, keto, South Beach and Atkins—can be quite expensive, as they emphasize pricey items like wild salmon, grass-fed beef, free-range chicken and organic produce. Vegetarian, vegan, Mediterranean and WW diets allow more affordable foods like beans and lentils.

You Enjoy an Adult Beverage

You can replace the cream in your coffee with skim milk, but there's no swap for a glass of wine or cocktail. If you want an occasional drink, avoid a teetotal plan.

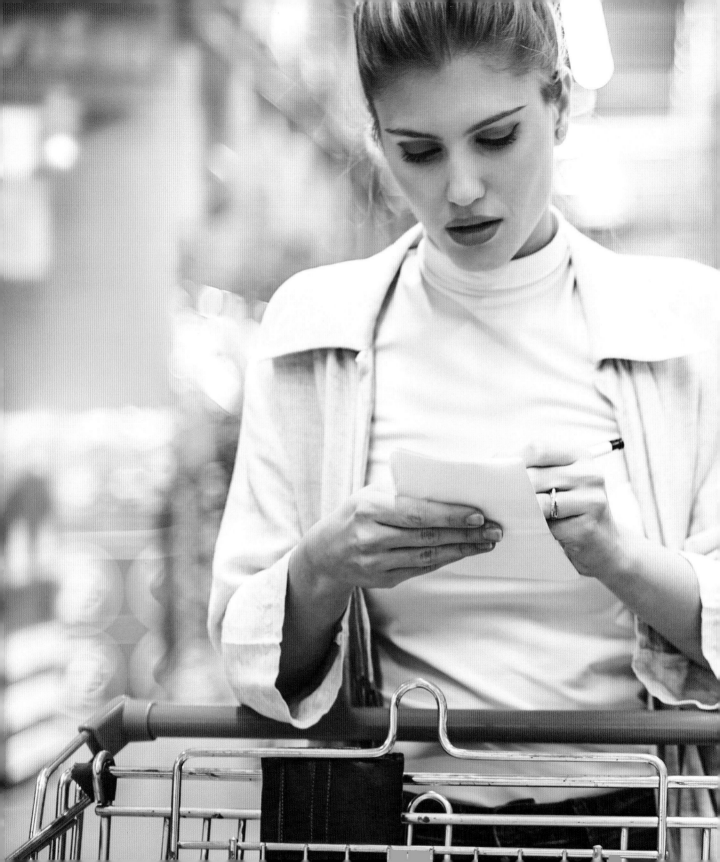

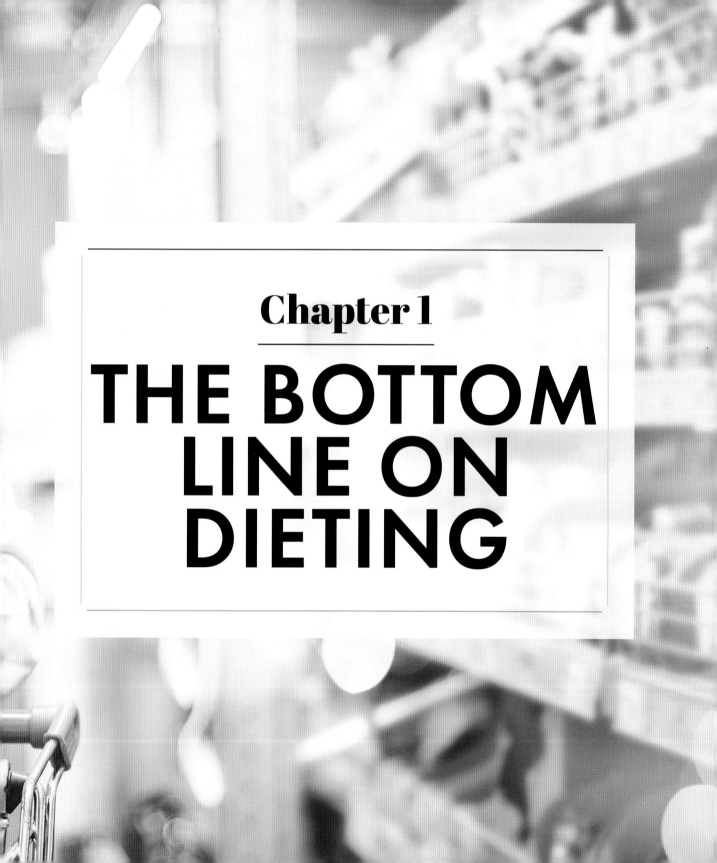

Chapter 1

THE BOTTOM LINE ON DIETING

What Drives Our Diet Obsession

Despite decades of ever-changing weight-loss methods being invented, obesity rates are still stubbornly climbing—and there's no shortage of dieters. Here, a few reasons people give for wanting to shed pounds.

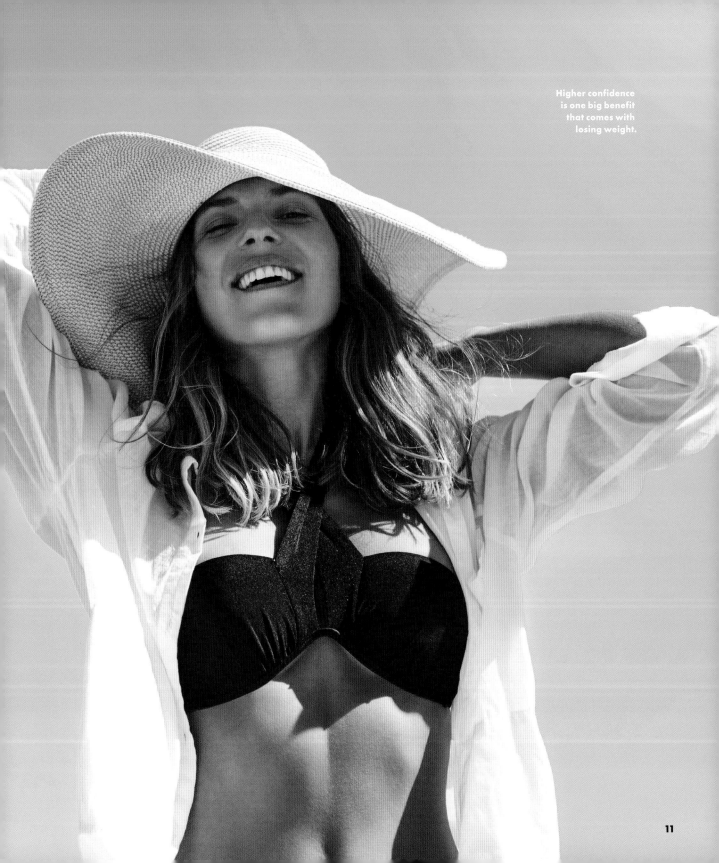

Higher confidence is one big benefit that comes with losing weight.

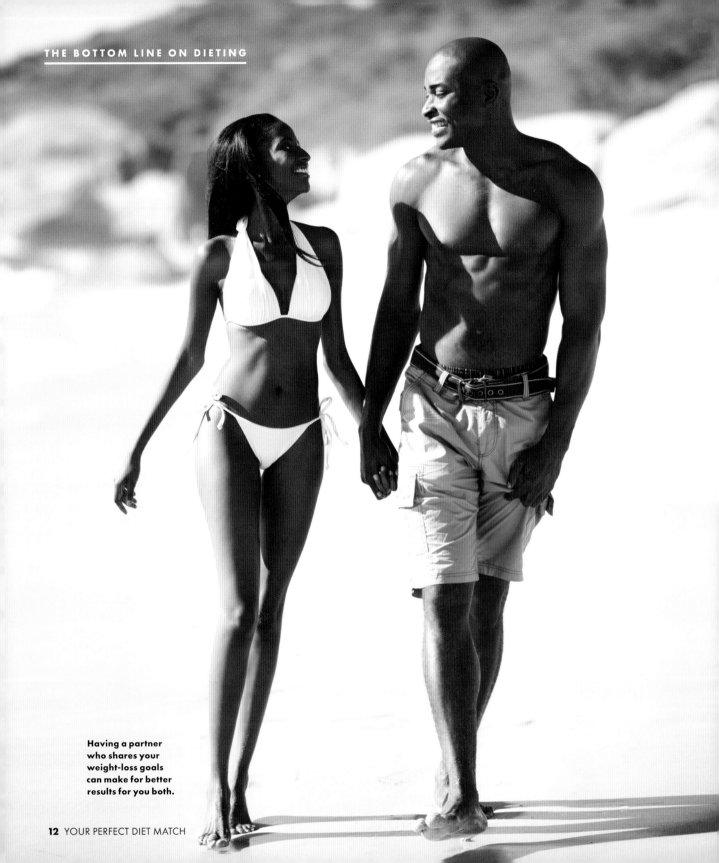

Having a partner who shares your weight-loss goals can make for better results for you both.

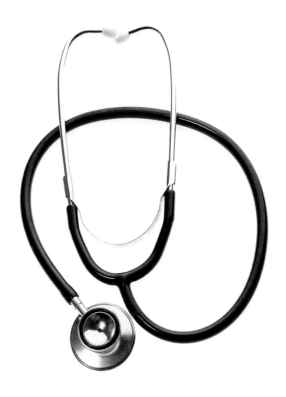

We live at a time plagued by unprecedented obesity rates, with many Americans living at unhealthy weights. Despite heightened awareness of the issues at root, new statistics are alarming—the latest government data reveals some 100 million Americans are now obese.

It seems that despite our nation's hyper-awareness of how sick and tired we are (scenes from *The Biggest Loser* and *My 600-lb. Life* come to mind), the struggle is still very real. Societal pressures to just "get skinny already"—coupled with the need to improve dire health issues linked to excess heft—have helped to fuel an obsession with dieting as a means to slim down. And although decades of restricted eating haven't gotten us anywhere, we're somehow still desperate to diet. Here, experts share what they hear as the main reasons so many of us continue to go on diets.

Feel Better

"People who come to see me tell me they just don't feel well," says Mimi Guarneri, M.D., cardiologist and president of the Academy of Integrative Health & Medicine. "They're tired and sluggish." Many times, she adds, they're in pain and experiencing side effects of lugging around excess weight—like sore backs and achy knees. More than just the pain, their confidence is shot. They feel bad that their clothes no longer fit and aren't happy with the way they look. "As for feeling better, just adding more walks to your day will have you smiling more right away," Guarneri says—definitely more than severely slashing calories, which can leave you irritated, weak, foggy and tired.

Unleash My Real Self

Unhappiness surrounding body image is probably the main reason people come to see Alexis Conason, Psy.D., a NYC–based psychologist who says most of her work is helping people overcome destructive body image and overeating. "People say they want to feel better about themselves and put themselves out there for a promotion or a date. Sometimes they want to be able to do things they've never done before and there's this fantasy that if they [lose the weight] they can become different people." But often, she says, people who think like this find that when they lose the weight, the things they hoped would happen...don't. "They're still not happy," she says. Conason tells her patients that the solution is changing their mindset and not dieting. "Body image is something that can be improved at any size," she says. Tune out the negative voice within.

Qualify for Bariatric Surgery

One of the more recent reasons patients tell Wilnise Jasmin, M.D., that they want to diet, along with wanting to relieve sleep apnea and ease painful osteoarthritis, is that they want to qualify for bariatric surgery. "This is one of the

Following a set eating plan can help you take control of your caloric intake.

main concerns I hear about," she says. Although most patients need to be at least 100 pounds overweight in order to qualify for weight-loss surgery, on the other end of the spectrum, it can be easier and safer to perform a bariatric operation if the patient has begun a reduced-calorie diet and started working out to lose weight. Jasmin tells patients "studies have shown that there is no one-size-fits-all approach and that no one diet outperforms others." Instead of dieting, she recommends making small daily changes that can permanently alter the way you eat, such as preparing meals at home, limiting processed and fried foods, and skipping the takeout.

Feel in Control

The desire to diet may also stem from a desire to take charge, says Conason. Some of her patients fear that if they don't follow a diet plan, they'll be tempted to overeat and consume all the foods they shouldn't. While some seek out diets as a way to gain control over their bodies, temptations and lives, "the ironic thing is that the more diets and strict rules we place on ourselves, the more out of control we feel," says Conason. "It's like a Chinese finger trap."

Instead of dieting, develop a more loving relationship with yourself, eat in a way that fosters that, and find ways other than food to nurture emotional needs, Conason advises. "It's not about being perfect; it's about being compassionate toward ourselves," she says.

Reverse This Health Issue

Often, patients referred to Guarneri's practice have been sent by their physicians because of a health scare, like developing an increased risk for heart disease, or a chronic condition such as Type 2 diabetes. Sometimes they've been living with the condition and are ready to get off their medications. "I see people get very motivated by being sick with risk factors for heart disease," says Guarneri. "They're suffering from things like sleep apnea, Type 2 diabetes, high blood

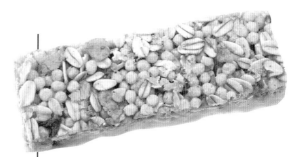

HOW THE DIET INDUSTRY IS CHANGING

• It may surprise you that the number of dieters in the U.S. has actually fallen in recent years. However, at the same time, industry revenue has shot up—with the U.S. weight-loss market as a whole still raking in about $66 billion annually.

• "The word 'diet' has a negative connotation now," says Mimi Guarneri, M.D. According to a December 2017 study by Marketdata, the number of U.S. dieters has dropped 10 percent since 2015 (though there are still nearly 100 million dieters).

• Another reason for the drop in dedicated dieters is the "fat acceptance movement." This movement is aimed at eliminating discrimination and helping large people live with dignity.

• Shakes and nutrition bars are still selling well; this may be because many Americans try to lose weight on their own.

• Online diet programs are increasingly popular —and lucrative, valued at $1 billion.

• The good news is that demand for prescription obesity drugs hasn't increased. But bariatric surgery is booming, with over 228,000 Americans going under the knife in 2017.

• A focus on health and wellness is predicted to be the next big thing. For those who believe it's actually blissed-out yogis who have all the fun, it's about time.

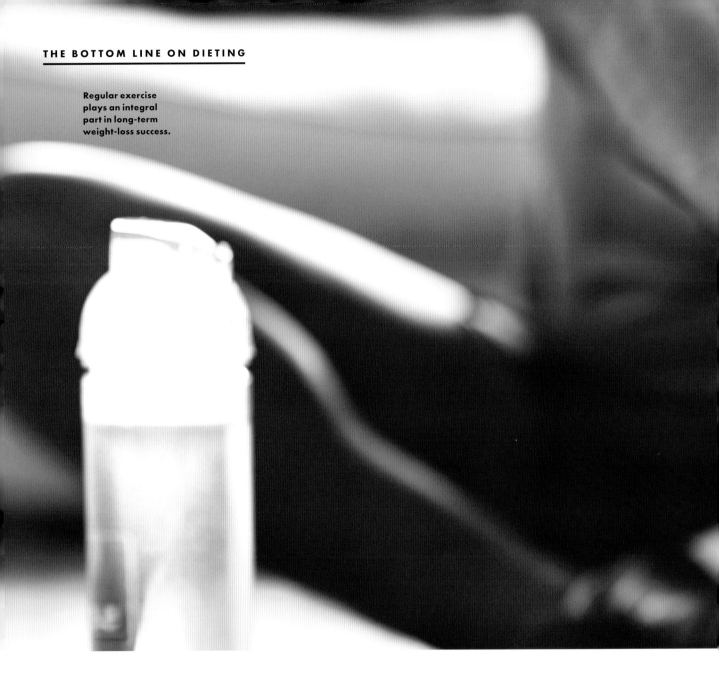

Regular exercise plays an integral part in long-term weight-loss success.

pressure, and high cholesterol—and they realize if they don't do something, they're going to be in real trouble."

The good news is that you can reverse heart disease and significantly improve diabetes, fatty liver, osteoporosis and other chronic diseases by making lifestyle changes. Those include eating a healthier diet and getting regular exercise, as well as addressing underlying issues, from depression to stress to heavy drinking.

Do Things I Love Again

While she admits some clients just want to look better, getting back to hiking or playing with

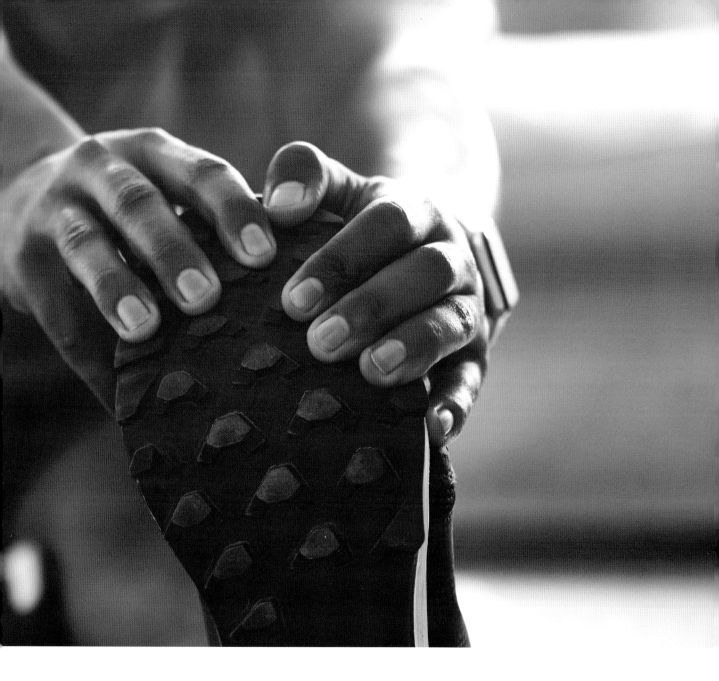

their grandkids are also common reasons folks see Virginia-based Jill Weisenberger, M.S., R.D.N., who wrote *Prediabetes: A Complete Guide*. "There's nearly always some emotion tied to a client's decision to seek my expertise," says Weisenberger. "I commonly see people who have spent years trying to lose weight with only temporary success." She works with her clients to kick extreme dieting measures to the curb while learning about healthful eating and all the steps they need to go through to find real, lasting results. "Those who have the most success with me are willing to move slowly through the whole process," she says.

**Struggling with
weight loss?
Your brain may
play a big part.**

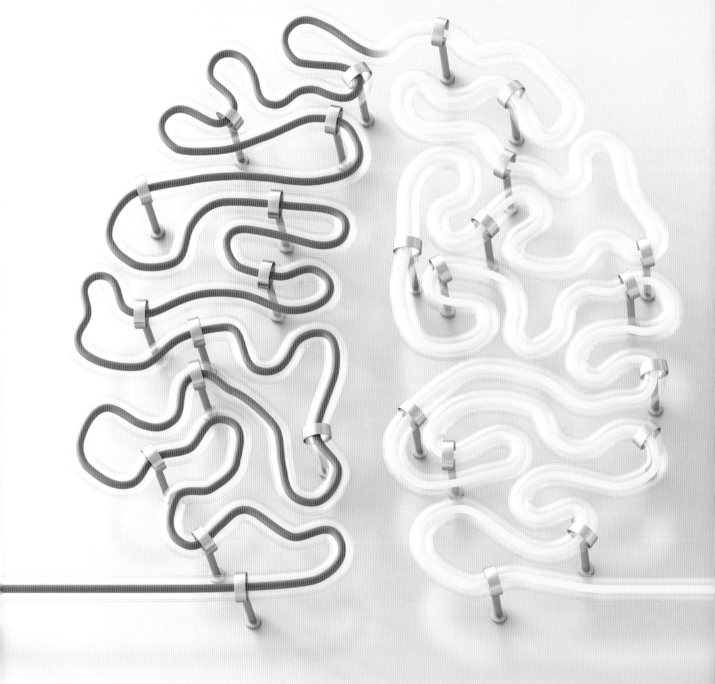

Why Dieting Really Is All in Your Head

*Discover how to train your mind
so you can shed pounds for good.*

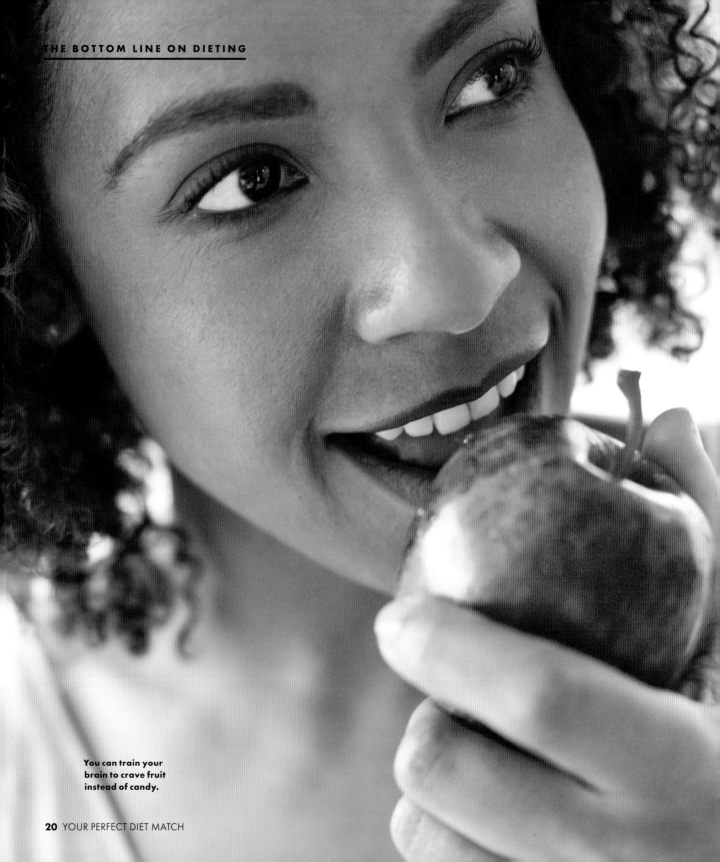

You can train your
brain to crave fruit
instead of candy.

In the battle to lose weight, your brain often conspires against you. Each day, we make an estimated 200 decisions about what we're going to eat. And every image, mention or smell of food sets off a complicated decision-making process in your mind, as well as a complex physical reaction to that food cue. So if you suddenly find yourself picking up a candy bar at the checkout counter, it's not that you lacked willpower—your brain was simply acting on impulse.

For years, diet experts believed that hunger and satiety were based in the body and that someone who struggled with their weight simply didn't have enough self-control to stay away from unhealthy foods. But thanks to new advances in neuroimaging, scientists are finally beginning to understand the role that different regions in the brain play when it comes to making important decisions about what we eat. And as research advances, the paradigm of weight loss being about personal choice continues to unravel.

Today, experts better understand that eating is the result of neurological, habitual and hormonal processes—not just simple physical hunger cues (although those do play a part). MRI imaging has identified strong reactions in the important, decision-making portions of the brain related to things like rewards and inhibitory control.

Of course, all brains are not created equal— which leaves some of us with more persistent, constant cravings and perceived hunger than others. The good news? Your brain can be retrained, says Susan B. Roberts, Ph.D., a professor of nutrition and psychiatry at Tufts University and founder of the iDiet weight-loss program, which works to retrain your brain to make healthier choices.

How We Got Here

Humans evolved while living in a highly food-deprived environment for a significant part of our existence. And while some areas of the world still struggle with a lack of accessibility to food, most of us don't have to worry about hunting or gathering to get supper on the table. In fact, our brains' underlying human drive to survive has collided with a rapid evolution of immediately accessible food.

Understanding that the brain has not evolved as quickly as the environment around us is an important piece of the puzzle. Those old neurological impulses and responses to seek food, crave food and eat all the food we can find are still in overdrive. And in our food-obsessed culture, where we are constantly surrounded by tantalizing ads, delicious smells and tempting goodies, they can actually undermine our health.

Brain Battles

Three distinct neurological processes are thought to be at the heart (brain) of our battle with food: the reward center, inhibitory control and our love of immediate gratification. It is easy to understand that the reward centers in our brains respond with a dose of dopamine (that happiness brain chemical) when we give in to sugary food cravings. But how do we short-circuit those responses? The choice to eat when we know we are not hungry is an intense struggle between the reward center and an effort in the prefrontal cortex to exhibit control, according to an article by neuroscientists published in the *Journal of the American Dietetic Association*.

In the article, researchers from Rush University Medical Center in Chicago explained that our ability to maintain willpower is challenged when we've had to expend energy in other areas of self-control throughout the day. If you grow tired from other decision-making processes, you may find yourself searching out a reward with food— likely the high-fat, high-sugar kind. And anytime you grow stressed or are physically exhausted, your inhibitory control is reduced—which is why you're more likely to order a pizza for dinner, even though you had better intentions earlier in the day.

Our brains and bodies are doing just what they are supposed to do with those reactions, says Roberts. The brain wants to streamline all decision making, and relegate decisions you repeatedly make into habits. It wants the pleasant hit that a candy bar will bring, and the anticipation of that dopamine reward is a strong pull. Symptoms of this desire for a short-term reward are both physical—the mouth watering, the stomach grumbling—and emotional.

Experts agree that it's not all about self-control. "Willpower is a myth, and it simply doesn't work," notes Judson A. Brewer, M.D., Ph.D., director of research and innovation at the Mindfulness Center at Brown University. Brewer has developed an eating system and an app based on mindfulness studies and MRI scans that uncovered a key area in the brain, called the orbitofrontal cortex, that stores "reward value." His approach teaches participants to focus their efforts on building awareness about their choices and to tap into more intrinsic rewards (healthy foods, feeling better and self-compassion) rather than external reward mechanisms, like weighing oneself. "This works to redirect participants into the present moment and to become curious about their cravings and urges rather than following a restrictive food plan," he explains.

Establishing Healthy Habits

Taking a step back to think of eating as behavioral and cultural and as a result of the brain's impulses, habits and hormones provides an entirely new perspective on the science of weight loss. "Our brains are very good at creating habits," says Roberts. "Any consistent and repetitive choice can become the new habit." For instance, if you ate an apple each time you were hungry for a snack all week long, you could actually train your mind and body to crave the healthier choice.

Roberts' groundbreaking study at Tufts University found we can, in fact, change our brains to crave healthier foods through repetition. Her team used MRI technology to scan the brains of participants at the beginning and the end of a

HABIT CHANGES

Try one of these shifts this week to start retraining your brain.

• Add a fruit or vegetable to every meal or snack.

• Drink a glass of water before every meal.

• Brush your teeth when craving unhealthy foods.

• Force yourself to eat the healthier option first at mealtime, for a week or longer.

• Remove tempting treats from your home environment so you don't see them and get triggered.

• Skip watching commercials to reduce the amount of food images you are forced to see in a day.

• Bring lunch to work so you do not have to make another decision about food, thus keeping decision fatigue at bay.

• Try meditation through an app or on YouTube.

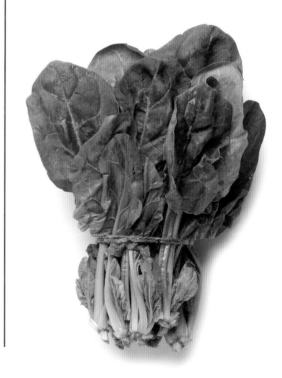

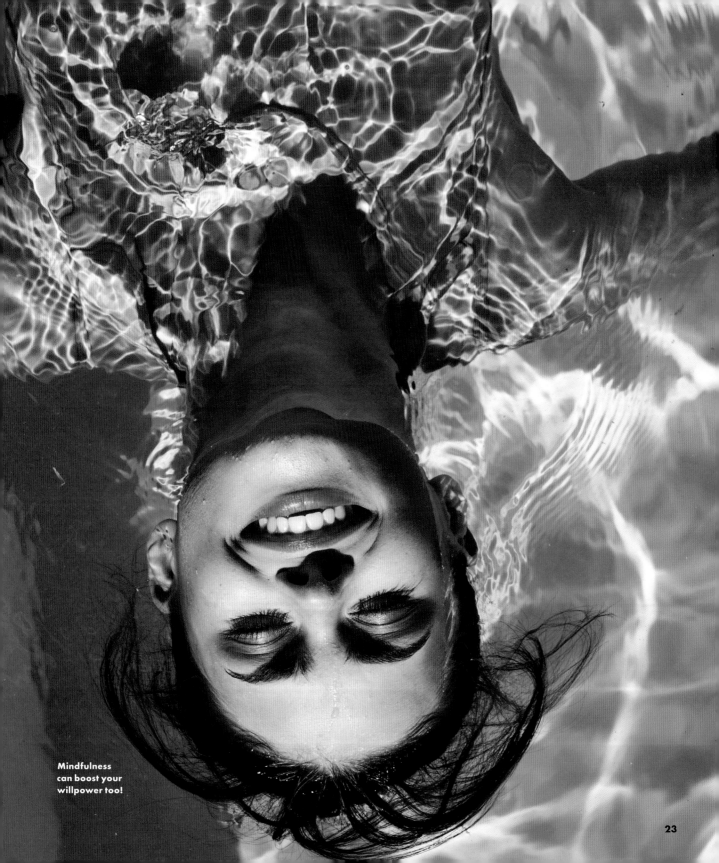

Mindfulness
can boost your
willpower too!

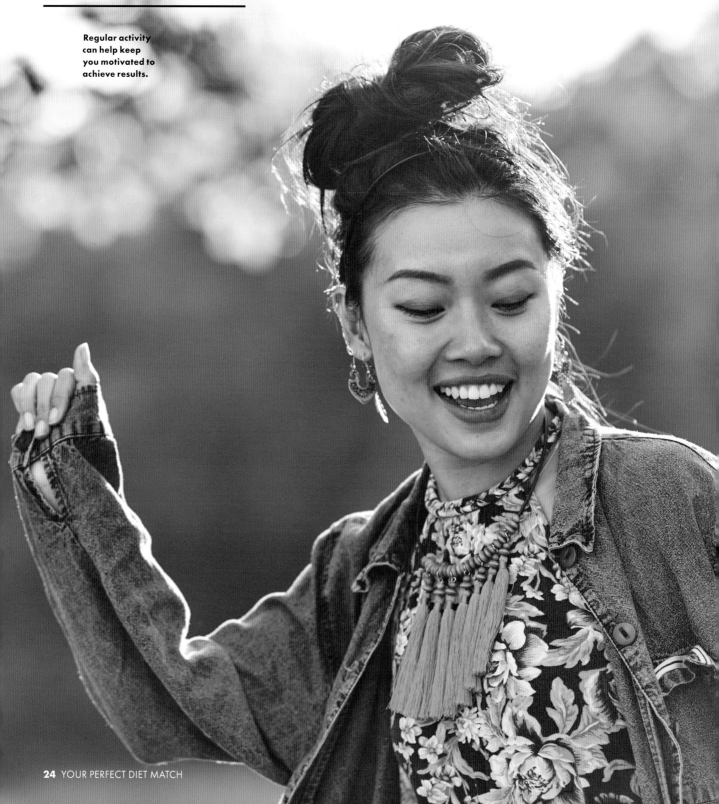

THE BOTTOM LINE ON DIETING

Regular activity
can help keep
you motivated to
achieve results.

six-month trial. By directing and supporting the participants to make healthier choices, researchers found that the brain responses to unhealthy food choices diminished, and the cravings for healthier food increased. After six months, changes in the brain's reward center tied to learning and addiction showed increased activity toward healthy, lower-calorie foods.

See It, Want It, Eat It

Through scientific-imaging studies, we know that seeing food—even in images—activates a portion of the prefrontal cortex linked to desire and motivation. This area of the brain is also responsible for stimulating hunger when the body is in a caloric deficit (or on a "diet").

When you restrict calories, the body sends hormone levels into a survival-mode shift. It increases the hormone ghrelin (that urges us to eat) and suppresses leptin (the hormone that tells us to stop eating), making us hungrier as we lose weight. In a sneaky shift to try and keep us alive, the brain urges overeating—and it seems as real as it feels.

As we begin to lose weight, research shows, the ventral medial prefrontal cortex responds less and less to pictures of food over time—with the decline in brain activity greatest among people who lost the most weight. On the other hand, activity in the lateral prefrontal cortex, involved in self-regulation, increased over the course of the diet. The more active it was, the more weight people lost. Bottom line: The longer you can stick with a healthier diet, the more your brain begins to crave those foods. And the more weight you lose, the more regulation seems to be activated. It's a cascading effect.

Keys to Success

Learning and using simple tricks and techniques to override the brain's impulses shows excellent results. The key is repetition, says Roberts. Anything done repeatedly and with consistency can become the new normal. For example, adding a fruit or vegetable to every meal or snack will take thought at first, but it will eventually become your new habit. Your palate will crave it over time.

With a better understanding of the brain, we're likely to see more and more effective weight-loss strategies. Science has already proven that exercising the brain in new ways where you're building the muscle of delayed gratification can yield results.

Using techniques like habit formation, gamification in the form of team challenges and reward systems, and even a gratitude practice can have promising outcomes as well. These strategies trick the brain into highlighting the same area that food does, creating new pleasure responses, and may normalize the intake of healthy foods. And that's something your brain —and body—can get behind.

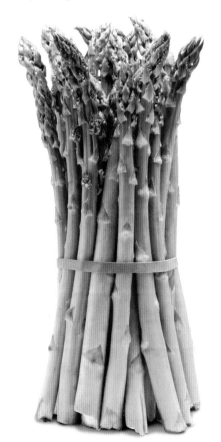

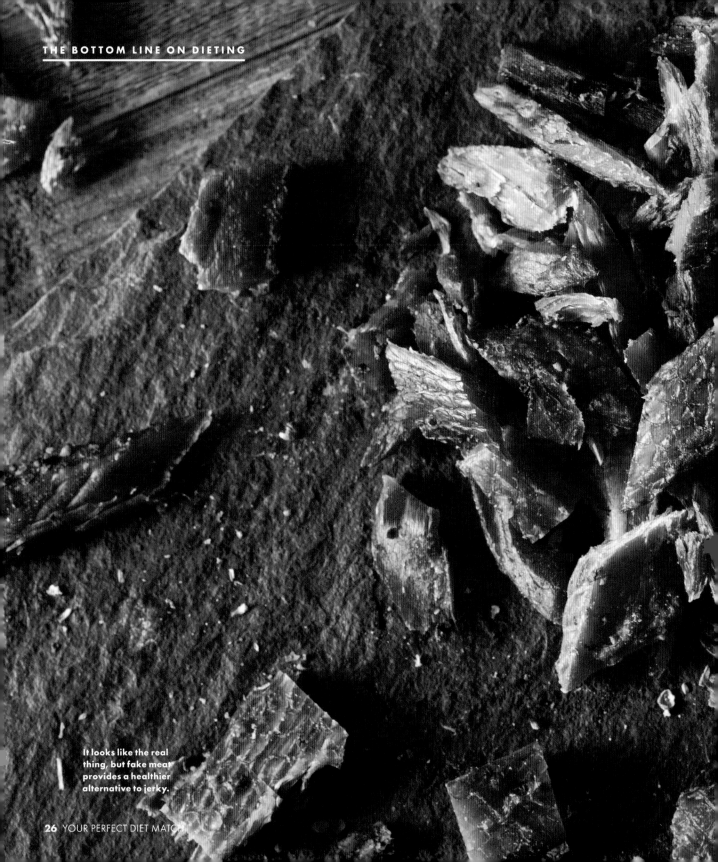

It looks like the real
thing, but fake meat
provides a healthier
alternative to jerky.

Top 10 Food and Diet Crazes Right Now

Learn all about the weight-loss and nutrition fads everyone is—or will soon be—talking about.

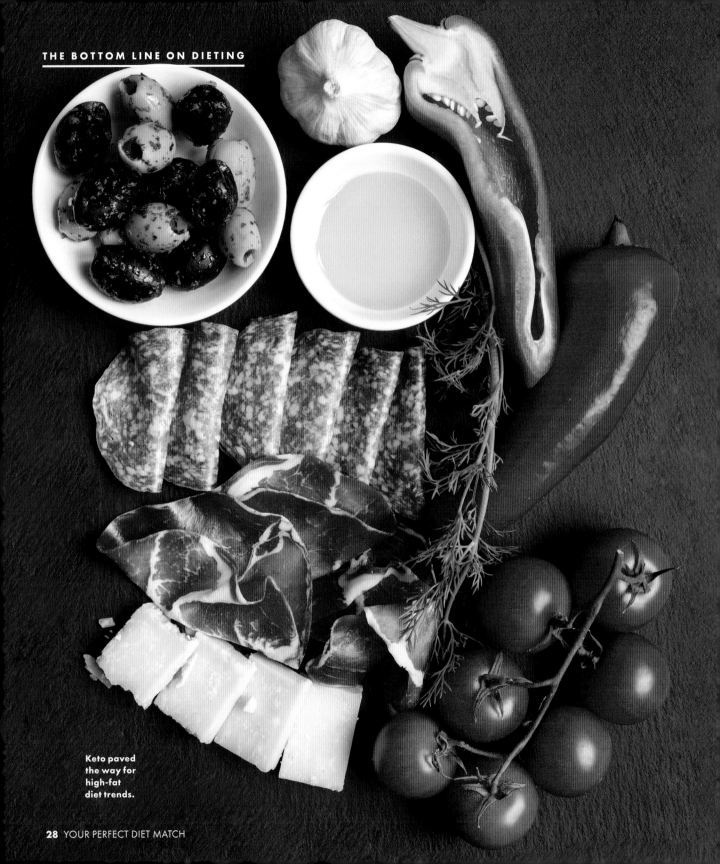

Keto paved
the way for
high-fat
diet trends.

U nicorn cake. Carnivore diet. Keto bread. These were just a few of the trending diet searches people typed into Google in the past couple of years. While most of these fads were fleeting—flooding Instagram feeds for a few months, only to be overtaken by the next craze—some have had the power to stick around (and no, we don't mean unicorn cake).

Keto and Paleo diets have piqued the interest of those looking to lose weight. They've shifted people's eating styles—favoring fats over carbs—and influenced the products hitting shelves. Alternatively, a shift toward plant-based eating has resulted in more meat alternative products, for both vegetarians and meat eaters alike.

Curious about what's ahead when it comes to new foods and diet trends? We tapped nutritionists and data from major supermarket chains for their list of predictions. Here's what you may find.

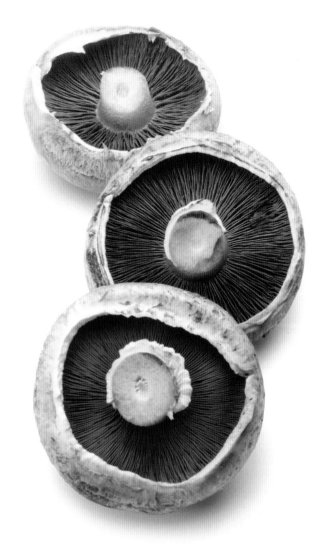

1 CBD Products

Cannabidiol (aka CBD) is a component of cannabis that won't get you high but it may help your health in a number of ways—including aiding weight loss. Some research shows it may help reduce appetite by blocking hunger receptors. You'll find CBD in an ever-growing variety of products, including coffees, seltzers and desserts.

2 Plant-Based Snacks

Faux jerky, pork rinds and bacon provide all the meaty texture and flavor you crave without any actual meat. Vegetarian and vegan foods aren't new to the scene, but consumer-trend experts say meat eaters are getting on board with vegetarian and vegan snacks and meals. And that's a good thing for both weight loss and health. "The benefits of plant-based foods include lower saturated fat and cholesterol intake and, generally, an increased fiber intake," says Jim White, R.D., a health and fitness specialist. Mushrooms are the star of this meat-free product

show. Their "meaty" texture makes them a satisfying, low-calorie alternative. You can find mushroom "jerky," mushroom-based gravies, breakfast patties and snacks.

3 Fats Are Back

"Once feared in our food culture, fats have grown in popularity due to the ketogenic diet," White says. Most are healthy in moderation—beneficial for increasing satiety, improving heart health and reducing inflammation. You'll see keto-friendly bars and portable nut-butter packs, made with MCT oil; "fat bombs" (coconut butter–filled chocolates);

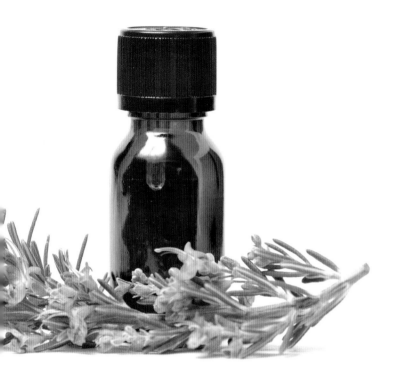

"And foods containing added prebiotic fiber—like chicory root, beans and Jerusalem artichoke—can be added to foods to feed gut bacteria." This all comes after an influx of research has illuminated the importance of healthy gut microbiomes to overall wellness. Healthy gut bacteria impact how food is digested and feelings of satiety, so they can aid in weight loss when everything is operating at peak performance. "Pre- and probiotics can be beneficial to digestion and immune health, and can aid some IBS sufferers," White adds. Just be careful with overconsumption, as too much can cause negative gastrointestinal symptoms including gas and bloating.

6 Anti-Added Sugars

Beginning in 2020, companies have been required to include added sugars on food labels, so you can expect some of the big names (like Nestlé, PepsiCo and General Mills) to keep tweaking formulas to appeal to customers, says White. Cutting back on added sugars can help you control your weight and lower your risk for certain diseases. Whole foods experts predict you'll see more monk fruit extract on food labels to replace added sugars.

7 Tahini Desserts

"Traditionally used in hummus, you'll notice tahini in desserts and sweet snacks as an alternative to peanut butter," White says. That's because tahini, made from sesame seeds, is safe for people with nut allergies. "It's high in calcium, vitamin E and B vitamins, as well as a good source of heart-healthy mono- and poly-unsaturated fatty acids." Studies have shown that diets high in monounsaturated fatty acids can help reduce belly fat. Keep portions in check if you're eating tahini desserts.

8 The Rise of Cabbage

If you stopped eating cabbage after trying the cabbage soup diet a few decades ago, it's time to find a place back on your menu for

and ready-to-drink vegan coffee inspired by butter coffees. The availability of these snacks makes it easier to follow a keto diet while traveling or any time you're away from home.

4 Essential Oils

Essential oils have been around for years and have known calming and stimulating effects, but according to *The Essential Oils Diet* by Eric Zielinski, D.C., their scents may also aid in dieting. Most essential oils need to be diluted for topical application, or they can be inhaled, but many should not be consumed. Research shows that inhaling grapefruit oil or cinnamon oil may help reduce appetite and cravings.

5 Gut-Friendly Foods

"More probiotic drinks, bars, dairy alternatives, nut butters, soups and cereals will be trending [in coming years]," says White.

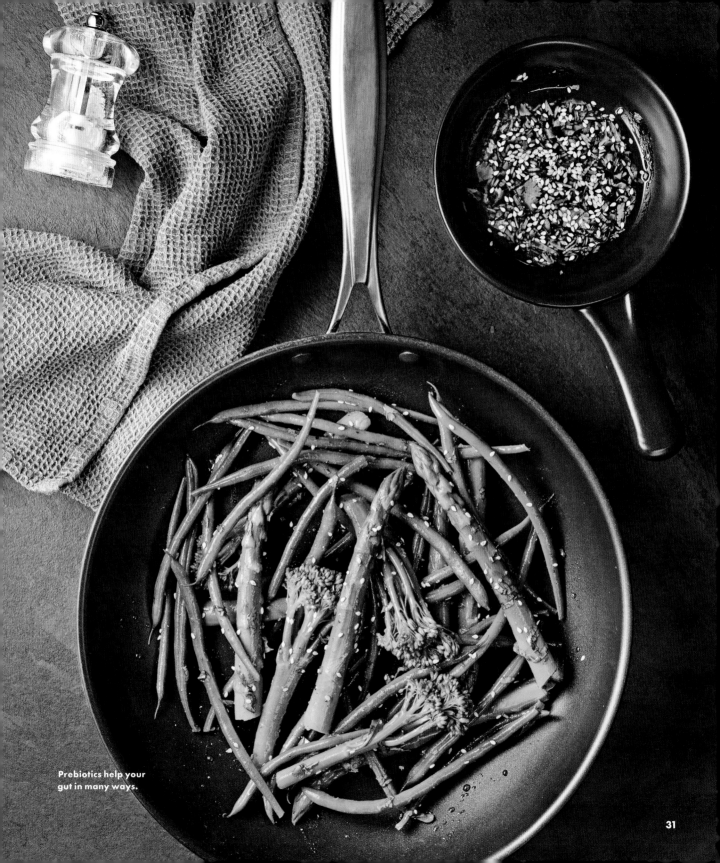

Prebiotics help your gut in many ways.

31

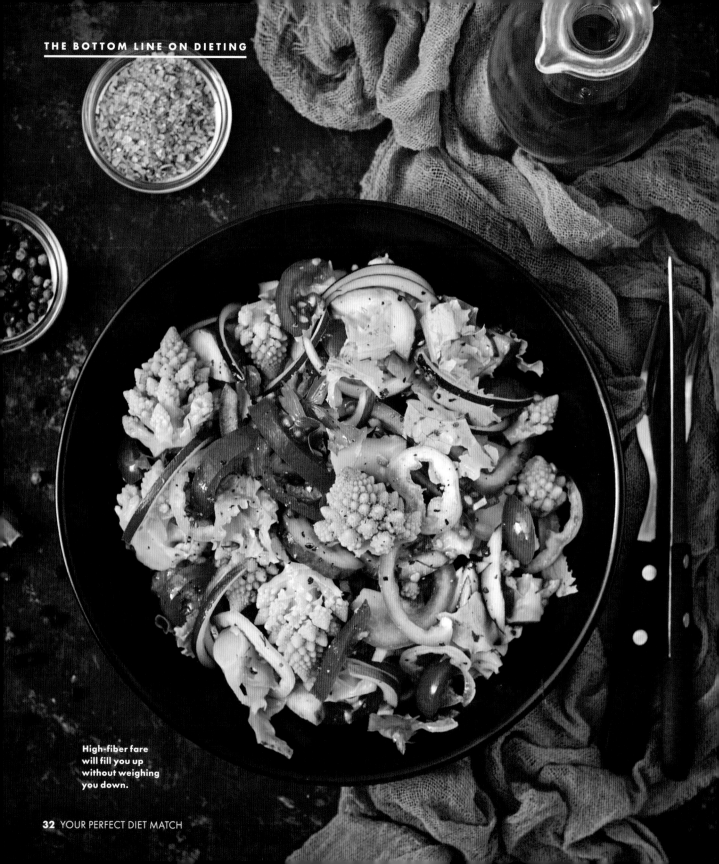

High-fiber fare
will fill you up
without weighing
you down.

this cruciferous vegetable. "Similar to cauliflower, cabbage will be all the rage as a low-carb option, replacing tortillas, wraps and noodles in a variety of dishes," White predicts. High in vitamins C and K and fiber, and with only 2.4 grams of carbs for one cup, low-carb diet followers are increasingly incorporating the veggie into a variety of recipes and meals.

9 Seafood

"Ocean-inspired foods, like salmon skin, seaweed butter, kelp noodles and salmon jerky, are on the rise as trendy, healthier alternatives to common snack foods," White says. Branch out beyond prepackaged seaweed snacks to incorporate these foods into your diet. They can be good for your waistline, since many are low in calories and carbs but are packed with vitamins and nutrients.

10 Pacific Inspiration

Flavors from Asia, Oceania and the western parts of North and South America are infiltrating foods and snacks. Ingredients like longganisa (a Filipino pork sausage), dried shrimp, cuttlefish and shrimp paste are popping up on more menus, while fruits such as guava, dragon fruit and passion fruit are making their way into colorful smoothie bowls and cocktails. Jackfruit may dominate as a meat alternative. Using these foods wisely in your diet can help with weight loss if you go a more natural route and avoid fried dishes. Tailor the foods you try to your specific diet. Keto and Paleo diet followers might enjoy the variety of flavors found in the longganisa, while someone on a smoothie diet may want to add more exotic fruits to their drinks. Many of these Asia-Pacific tropical fruits are also available in the frozen fruits section as purees. Using dried shrimp and cuttlefish is a great way to add a lot of flavor to sauces and stir-fries with zero grams of fat and not a lot of calories. Apply these techniques if you're following a WW or Noom diet plan.

TASTE THE TRENDS

Try one of these swaps this week to start retraining your brain.

THE CRAZE Plant-Based Snacks/ Gut-Friendly Foods
TRY Plant-Based, Dairy-Free Lavva Yogurt

THE CRAZE Anti-Added Sugars
TRY Lakanto Monkfruit Sweetener

THE CRAZE Seafood
TRY Sea Tangle Noodle Company's Kelp Noodles, Ocean's Halo Sea Salt Seaweed Sheets

THE CRAZE Fats Are Back
TRY FBOMB Macadamia Pecan Nut Butter

THE CRAZE Pacific Inspiration
TRY The Jackfruit Company's Complete Jackfruit Meals

THE CRAZE CBD Products
TRY Tree Below Zero Sparkling Beverages

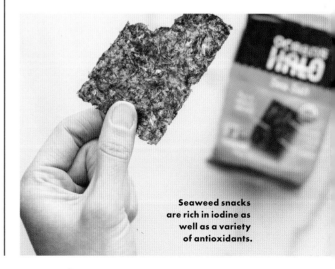

Seaweed snacks are rich in iodine as well as a variety of antioxidants.

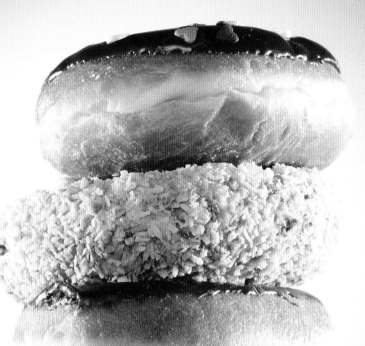

THE TRUTH ABOUT LOW-CARB DIETS

How these plans became popular, and how you can incorporate healthy options into your life.

Almost as popular as disco music, women's rights and *Star Wars* in the 1970s was the theory that dietary fat caused heart disease. Inspired by studies underscoring the negative impact of saturated fat upon cardiovascular health, the 1977 Federal Dietary Guidelines recommended capping dietary fat at 30 percent of daily energy intake and increasing carbohydrate intake to 60 percent. By the 1980s, low-fat diets had become cultural and medical gospel, influencing consumer behavior and food companies' marketing strategies.

The Low-Fat Paradox

"Ideally, lower-fat diets would have included vegetables, high-fiber fruits and whole grains," says Julie Stefanski, R.D.N., a spokesperson for the Academy of Nutrition and Dietetics and owner of Stefanski Nutrition Services. "But food manufacturers created highly processed, low-fiber and high-sugar items touted as 'healthy' because they were fat-free." Seduced by these products' sweetness and convinced that munching zero-fat snacks would spare their hearts—and waistlines—consumers gobbled them up, Stefanski says.

Cut to the early 2000s, when evidence refuting the link between high fat intake and risk of heart disease burst the anti-fat fervor's bubble. Fat, it turned out, was not the enemy. Saturated fat never proved itself to be strongly beneficial to health. But mono- and polyunsaturated "healthy" fats can improve "good" cholesterol levels, lower heart disease risk and help preserve cognition.

Simultaneously, all that consumption of fat-free, high-sugar, high-carb "health" foods appeared to be making Americans' disease prospects (and weight problems) worse. Studies linking excess consumption of sugar to heart disease, diabetes and obesity underscored this connection. Soon enough, carbohydrates usurped fat as the least-likable macronutrient.

Enter the low-carb diet craze. Consumers love these diets for the fast weight loss and reduced belly fat results they produce, while researchers are discovering a positive link between moderately low-carb diets and lower heart disease risk, as well as reduced blood sugar and insulin levels.

The Logic Behind Going Low

Clinical endorsement for low-carbohydrate diets dates back to the 1920s, when doctors prescribed "ketogenic diets"—allowing only 20 grams of carbs per day—to mitigate symptoms of epilepsy by reducing excitatory nerve impulses in the brain. In the late 20th century, the Atkins, South Beach and Paleo diets followed suit, with their own variations on low-carb lifestyles; each gained steam from the backlash against carbs following the fat-free faux pas. Their main selling point? Severely restricting carbohydrates (which the body breaks down into glucose) forces the body to tap into fat stores for fuel—a process called ketosis that can lead to weight loss.

As low-carbohydrate diets proved themselves to be effective in managing diabetes symptoms, enthusiasm for them grew. Anecdotal reports of pounds shed in the double—even triple—digits from those who adopted them also helped. No sooner had "fat-free" been struck from diet-food marketing tactics than "low-carb" took its coveted place.

Choose the "Right" Kind of Carbs

Carbs are considered to be either simple or complex. Simple carbs have chemical structures that are easily dismantled and absorbed into our bloodstream, like sucrose (in table sugar), fructose (in fruit) and lactose (in milk). Complex carbohydrates (think: starches and fiber) take longer to move from the digestive tract to the bloodstream. Complex carbohydrates offer longer-lasting energy and are associated with better health outcomes.

To reap the maximum health and weight-loss benefits, look to swap out simple carbs with less nutritional value (like white flour, pasta and bread) for healthier, complex carbs (like whole grains) as well as low-carb vegetables or fruits for fiber, vitamins and nutrients.

Changes in food labels better highlight additives and serving sizes.

The New Food Labels Guide

Here are the latest updates you'll see on packaged food products to help you make wiser choices.

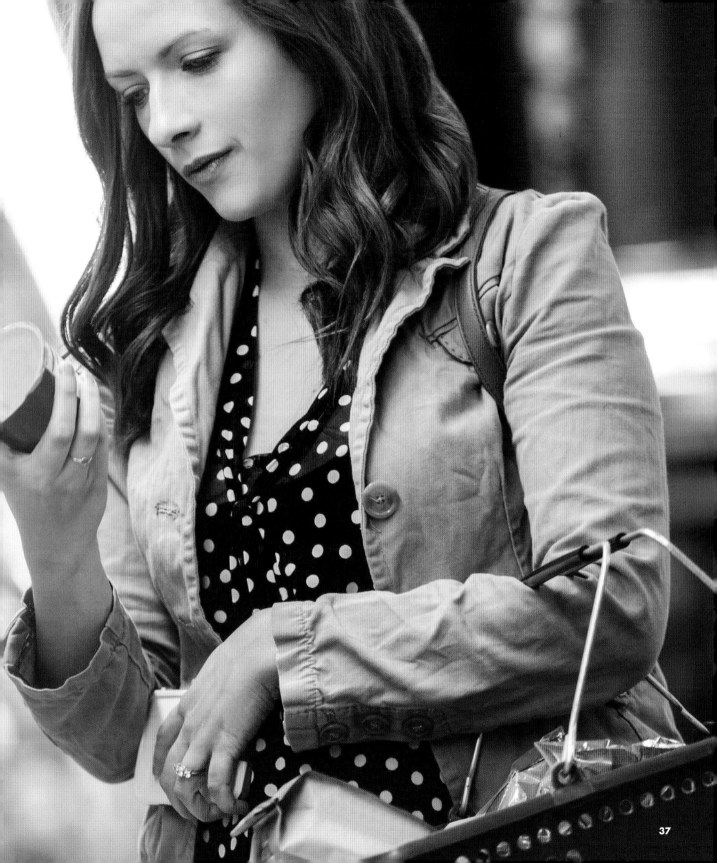

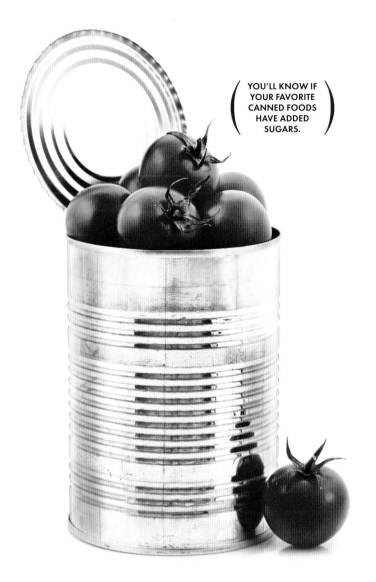

YOU'LL KNOW IF YOUR FAVORITE CANNED FOODS HAVE ADDED SUGARS.

Large companies had to make their changes by January 1, 2020; every other food company must have labels updated by January 1, 2021.

Here, Amy Gorin, M.S., R.D.N., and owner of Amy Gorin Nutrition in the New York City gives us the scoop on the new nutrition labels.

Serving Sizes & Easy-to-Read Information

Calories, servings per container, and serving size will be in larger, bolder type, making it easier for the consumer to see the information—and to make healthier food choices and save time while shopping, says Gorin.

Packaged-food serving sizes are being updated to reflect the portion that people often eat, based on the Nutrition Labeling and Education Act's established reference amounts, says Gorin. Some examples of changes that were made: A yogurt serving changed from 8 ounces to 6, and an ice cream serving is ⅔ cup, versus ½ cup. Some portions are decreasing while others are increasing, but "I'd still recommend you eat the ½-cup serving of ice cream to keep it to 143 calories for chocolate ice cream, versus 191 calories for a ⅔ cup serving," Gorin says.

Some small packages have multiple servings per container—which can make food decisions confusing for the consumer, says Gorin. The new label's information shows total servings per container; plus, for smaller containers, such as a pint of ice cream, you'll get "per serving" information as well as "per unit" information. This will help you avoid diet derailers, like when you don't notice that a snack contains more than one portion and then eat the whole bag—and double the number of calories you meant to consume.

Added Sugars Listed

For the first time, "added sugars" are listed both in grams and as a Percent Daily Value (DV). Gorin says this is a good thing to educate consumers about. "Hopefully, this change will help consumers understand the difference between naturally

There are a lot more changes coming to your favorite packaged-food products—and they're good for the savvy consumer who wants to know more about what's in his or her food and make smarter decisions: The U.S. Food and Drug Administration (FDA) has updated the Nutrition Facts label for packaged foods to reflect scientific changes.

occurring sugar in milk or fruit, and added sugar, such as brown sugar or honey." It's still important to read the ingredients and look out for added sugars, including "healthy-" and "natural-" sounding ones like maple syrup, molasses and honey, she says. "This label change will help people meet the goal of getting less than 10 percent of daily calories from added sugar," says Gorin. And no matter what diet you're following, whether it's vegan, Paleo, the DASH diet or intuitive eating, limiting sugar is a key to success.

Nutrient Updates

Now you can also see nutrient amounts on the label; previously, just the DV, which is a hard concept for many people to grasp, was shown. (Also, the DV was based on a 2,000-calorie daily diet, more than what most dieters eat.) The amount of vitamin D and potassium in an item is now listed on the label, along with calcium and iron, all of which help you stay healthy while losing weight. "Total Fat," "Saturated Fat," and "Trans Fat" remain on the label, but "Calories from Fat" was removed, because research shows the type of fat is more important than the amount. "Also, look to see how much protein, healthy fat and fiber a food contains," says Gorin. "These nutrients will work to keep you satiated." The new label will also help you stick to the specific diet you're following, so you won't overdo carbs while on Paleo, for instance.

What's Different?

Nutrition Facts

1 8 servings per container
Serving size 2/3 cup (55g) 4

Amount per serving
Calories **230** 5

% Daily Value* 6

Total Fat 8g	**10%**
Saturated Fat 1g	**5%**
Trans Fat 0g	
Cholesterol 0mg	**0%**
Sodium 160mg	**7%**
Total Carbohydrate 37g	**13%**
Dietary Fiber 4g	**14%**
Total Sugars 12g	
Includes 10g Added Sugars	**20%**
Protein 3g	

2

Vitamin D 2mcg	10%
Calcium 260mg	20%
Iron 8mg	45%
Potassium 235mg	6%

3

* The % Daily Value (DV) tells you how much a nutrient in a serving of food contributes to a daily diet. 2,000 calories a day is used for general nutrition advice 7

1. SERVINGS: LARGER, BOLDER TYPE
2. NEW: ADDED SUGARS
3. CHANGE IN NUTRIENTS REQUIRED
4. SERVING SIZES UPDATED
5. CALORIES: LARGER TYPE
6. UPDATED DAILY VALUES
7. ACTUAL AMOUNTS DECLARED

THE NEW LABELS
ARE NOW
ON NEARLY
EVERY PACKAGED
GROCERY ITEM.

Don't Fall for It

WEIGHT-LOSS FADS OVER THE DECADES

Americans have been seeking fast fixes to drop pounds for more than a century. Here's a look back at some of the strangest—and unhealthiest— diets that have been popular since your great-grandmother's generation.

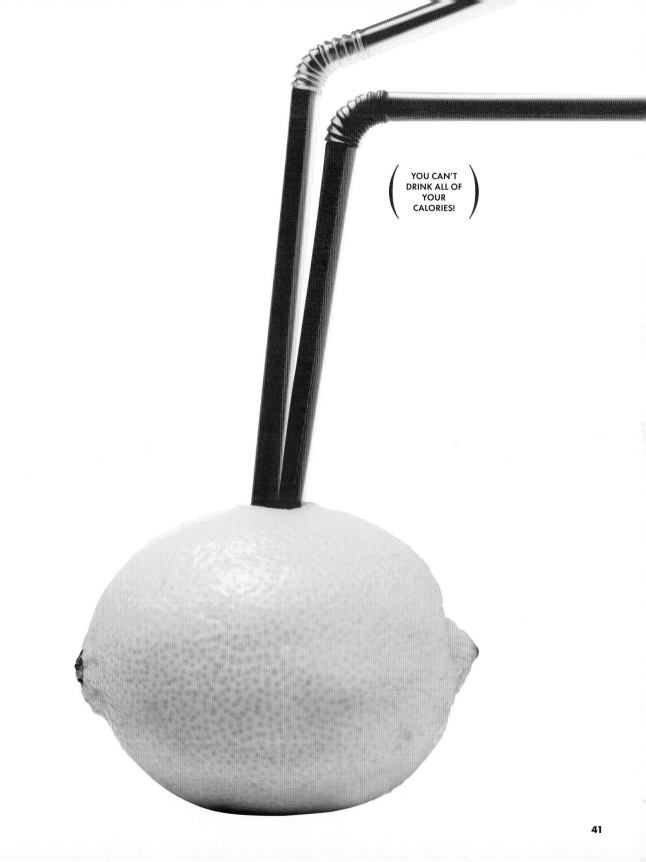

YOU CAN'T
DRINK ALL OF
YOUR
CALORIES!

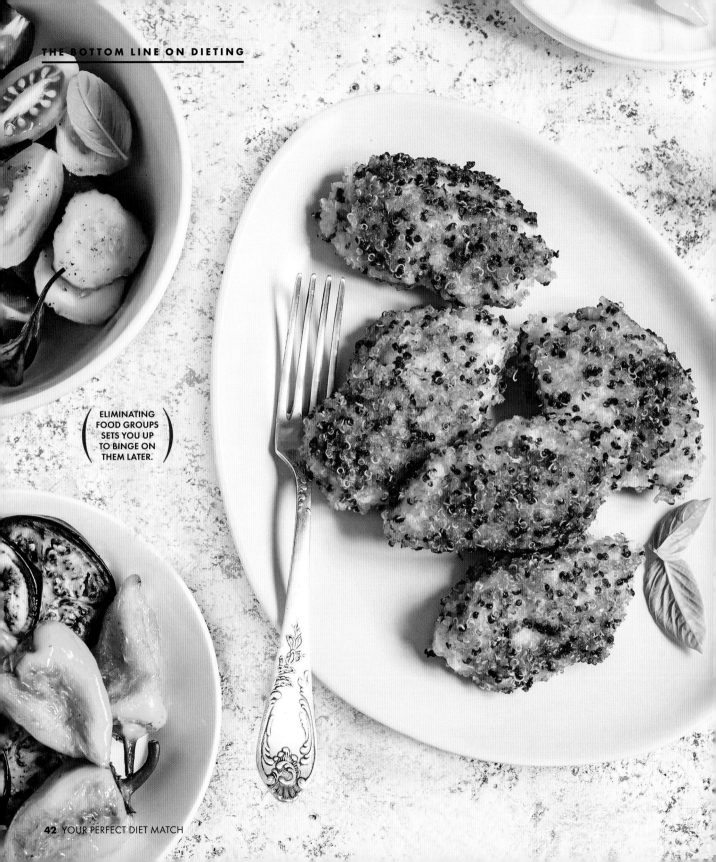

ELIMINATING
FOOD GROUPS
SETS YOU UP
TO BINGE ON
THEM LATER.

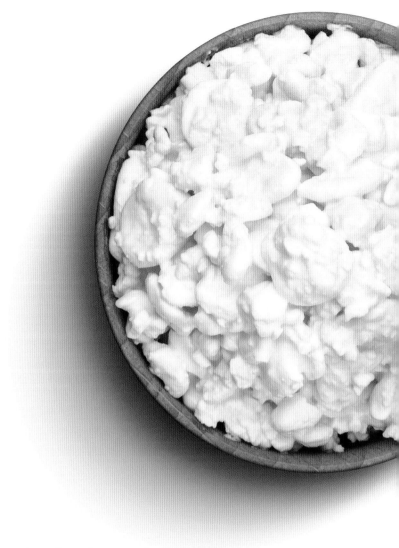

D ietary fads are nothing new. Evidence suggests that even ancient Egyptians and Mesopotamians fell for them. We may look back at historical dietary trends—like taking arsenic pills or willfully ingesting tapeworms to slim down—with shock and disgust. But around 97 million Americans still get ensnared by questionable approaches to weight loss each year. Fad diets' seductiveness lies in their "promise to quickly and easily wipe away our fears of being unattractive, getting older, or getting sick," says Kirsten David, M.S., R.D., an EduPlated dietitian. Here are nine diet fads Americans have fallen for over the past century.

1 Fletcherism

Promoted by self-proclaimed "economic nutritionist" Horace Fletcher in the early 1900s, Fletcherism advised masticating each bite of food to the point of liquefaction. "It was believed to boost digestion and improve oral hygiene," explains Steven Gundry, M.D., author of *The Plant Paradox*. "Weight loss usually followed…from the extended time it took to eat food; so naturally less was consumed."

2 Smoker's Diet

Fearing sales losses from proof that cigarettes were horrible for health, the tobacco industry reframed smoking as a weight-loss tool in the 1920s, suggesting that reaching for a smoke—instead of a snack—could shed pounds, Gundry explains. Sure, smoking in lieu of eating accomplished that. (Nicotine, the active ingredient in cigarettes, has been shown to increase metabolism in the short term.) But over the long haul, smoking is associated with weight gain—not to mention the increased risk of lung disease, heart disease and cancer.

3 Cottage Cheese Diet

The gist: A dish of cottage cheese for every meal and snack, though some versions allow spices, seasonings and occasionally fresh fruit and vegetables. "You may drop weight quickly, but you'll also deprive your body of essential macronutrients and micronutrients needed to function," cautions Michelle Routhenstein, M.S., R.D., founder of the nutrition counseling private practice Entirely Nourished. "You push your body into famine mode and risk reprogramming it to retain extra pounds once you start eating normally again," she says. That's a risk most fad diets entail. The cottage cheese diet began in the 1950s, but some people still follow it today.

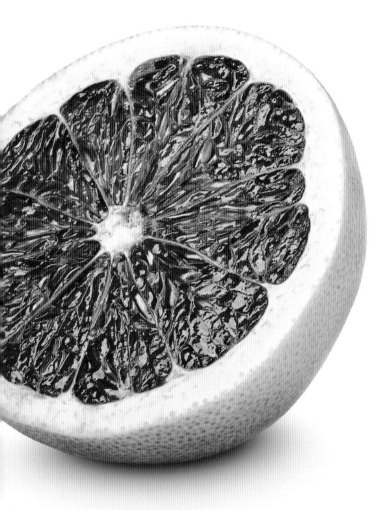

5 Grapefruit Diet

Enjoy the sweet tartness of fresh grapefruit? Now imagine eating it at every meal. That's the recommendation for this 12-day diet, whose dubious origins date back to the 1930s. In addition to having one half of a grapefruit and 8 ounces of grapefruit juice at each meal, adherents are allowed animal protein with breakfast, lunch and dinner, and a salad or vegetables with lunch and dinner. Minor detail: You restrict your daily caloric intake to under 1,000 calories (about half of what most people need to survive). Grapefruit's weight-loss effects have been shown to be no more powerful than the effect of drinking more water. So, why not eat healthfully and chug more H_2O?

6 The Blood Type Diet

In 1996, naturopathic doctor Peter D'Adamo pushed the idea that our blood type—A, B, AB or O—determines what we should eat to maintain optimal health. Type As, he proposed, should eat a more vegetarian diet; Bs should load up on dairy; ABs should combine those two approaches; and Type Os should eat more animal protein. Several studies have disproven the blood type diet's premise.

7 Fat-Free Diet

Remember when everyone was munching fat-free cookies and snacks because we thought fat was bad? This fear of fat started in the late 1970s but really took hold of Americans' dieting mindsets in the '90s. We began replacing foods that naturally contained fats with nonfat or low-fat options that were often highly processed and loaded with added sugar. And you know what happened? We got fatter. Shunning peanut butter, olive oil and avocados for fat-free cookies and plates of pasta didn't deliver the weight-loss results we thought it would—likely because cutting out fat can leave you feeling unsatisfied and hungry again after only a short time. Although some people still follow a low-fat diet, research now recognizes the

4 Cabbage Soup Diet

Promising to help you shed 17 pounds a week, this crash diet gained support from a small handful of doctors in the 1930s, '60s and '70s. Adherents eat a simmered cabbage head with celery and a slim range of other fixings as they want, plus one "specified" food that changes daily: fruits, vegetables, or a baked potato with butter, to name a few. Dietary experts say dropping pounds was mainly from water weight lost. Keep in mind, all that cabbage could make one quite gassy!

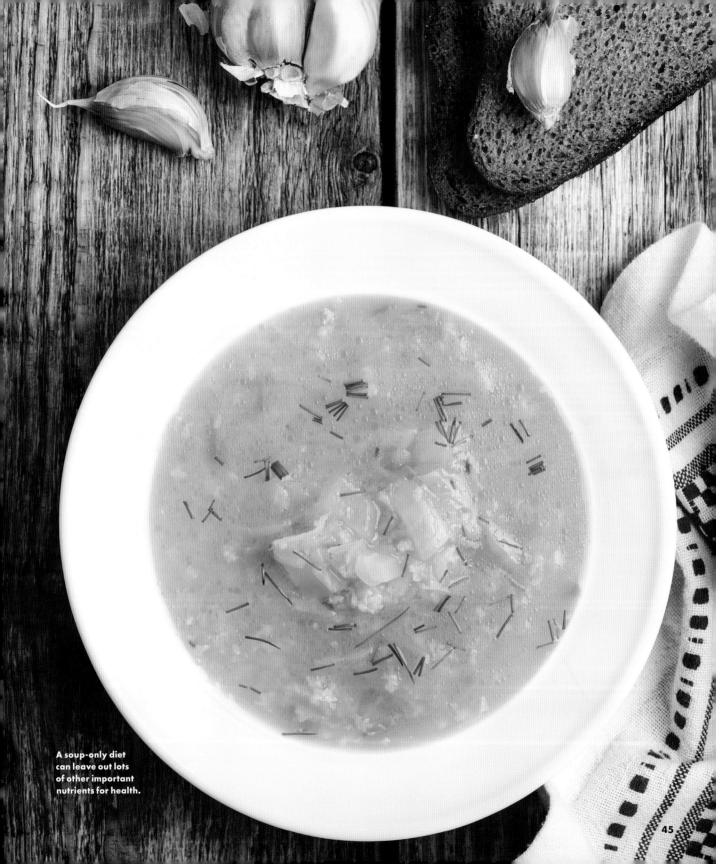

A soup-only diet can leave out lots of other important nutrients for health.

45

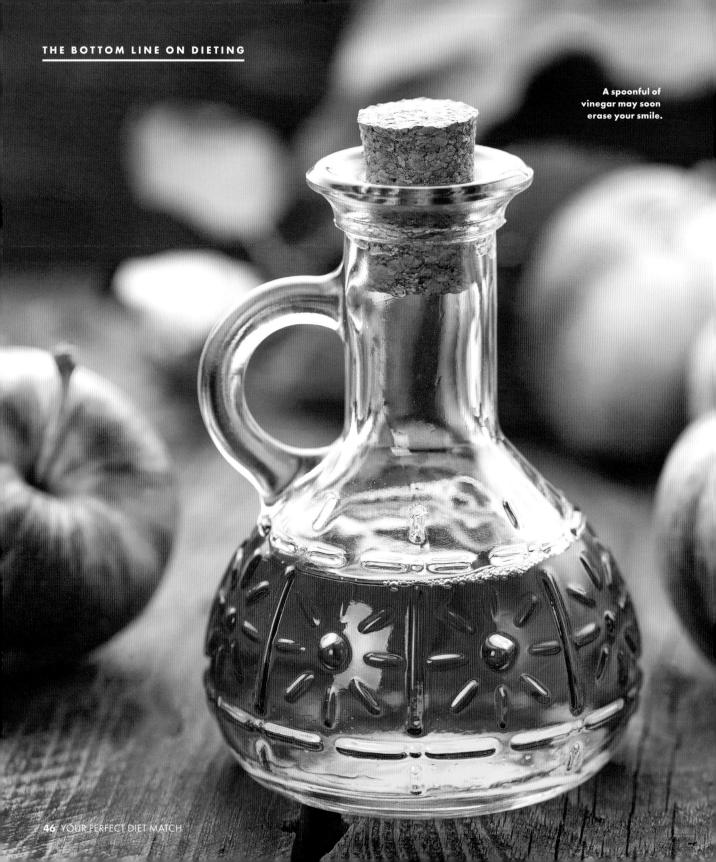

A spoonful of vinegar may soon erase your smile.

benefits of good (monounsaturated) fats in our diet, suggesting eating plans like the Mediterranean diet, which is based around foods that are naturally rich in healthy fats like nuts, fish and olive oil.

8 Apple Cider Vinegar Diet

You might be having a shot of apple cider because you've heard it can help with digestion and maybe even weight loss. Apple cider vinegar (ACV) is made when crushed apples go through a fermentation process, eventually turning into acetic acid—the active compound in vinegar. Some recommendations of the apple cider vinegar diet are to have 1 to 2 teaspoons of this liquid before or along with meals. This liquid has actually been around for centuries, but it's gained popularity as a weight-loss aid mostly within the past decade. Some studies have found that obese people who took ACV daily lost weight—but only 4 pounds over three months! Before you take on an ACV detox or cleanse, keep in mind that drinking this acidic supplement can erode tooth enamel and may cause negative digestive side effects—without the promise of significant weight loss.

9 Tapeworm Diet

Joking to a friend that you have a tapeworm because you're always hungry? This quip is actually misleading, because if you had a tapeworm, it would zap your appetite. Perhaps that's why the tapeworm diet came about in the early 20th century. Even though we should know better, one hundred years later some people have still tried this extreme tactic to lose weight. The tapeworm diet involves swallowing a pill that has a tapeworm egg inside, which hatches, grows inside your body, and eats whatever you're eating.

Health experts say that ingesting tapeworms is extremely risky and can cause a wide range of undesirable side effects, including—rarely—death. To get rid of the tapeworm, you'll need to get antibiotics from your doctor. We hope the days of this disgusting diet are long gone.

HOW TO SNIFF OUT A FAD

A 2006 review of bestselling diet-advice books found that a whopping 67 percent of nutrition facts cited in their pages is not supported by actual research. Beware these fad diet red flags:

• They promise rapid weight loss. You may notice your pants fitting a little looser if you stick to a fad diet for more than a week. But think twice before chucking your regular jeans for skinny versions, since one in six overweight dieters regain what they lose during a period of caloric restriction, according to studies.

• They suggest eliminating an entire food group. Or they warn that an entire food group will make you gravely ill. While some individuals are genuinely allergic to certain foods, it can be dangerous to nix an entire food group (say, all protein or all grains) from your diet.

• They promote a product. Tying a diet to a perfectly calibrated energy bar, a meticulously titrated supplement, or some other prepackaged goodie is a strong sign the diet founders are probably more interested in part of your paycheck than your health and weight goals.

• Their claims aren't based on peer-reviewed research in humans. Fact-check a diet's claims by looking up the references. If there aren't any, that's a red flag in and of itself.

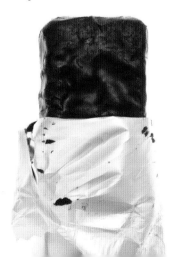

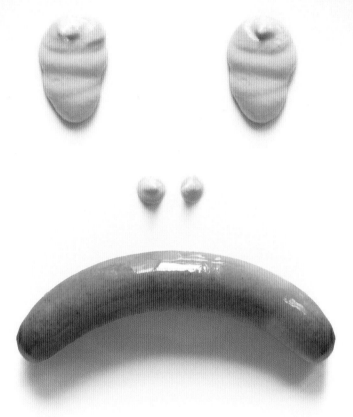

IF A PLAN SOUNDS TOO GOOD TO BE TRUE, IT PROBABLY IS.

THE 8 WORST DIETS EVER

Learn about the extreme lengths to which some have gone with fad weight-loss plans for rapid results—and the health toll they take.

About 45 million Americans diet each year—and for some, a fad diet's allure is too enticing to ignore. With straightforward rules, they appear easy to follow. "They're touted as quick fixes. But the weight crept on slowly and…it should come off slowly," says Anne VanBeber, Ph.D., R.D., professor and chair of the Department of Nutritional Sciences at Texas Christian University.

The swift weight loss is real, but so are the long-term health consequences. "Any weight-loss situation involving extreme calorie-cutting can be damaging hormonally," says Chicago-based Amanda Baker Lemein, R.D., M.S. Here, some of the wackiest diets that have seduced us.

1 HCG Diet

Claims of slashing up to 30 pounds in 30 days had thousands of dieters sticking syringes of hCG (human chorionic gonadotropin) in their thighs while starving themselves. It's not only ineffective—it can be extremely harmful, says Lemein.

2 Gluten-Free Diet

Back in the 1940s, a pediatrician noted that a wartime wheat-free diet helped children with celiac disease. Those on gluten-free diets today skip gluten, a protein found in wheat, barley, rye and other grains. But there is no proof that people without celiac disease, wheat allergies or gluten sensitivity will lose weight or gain health benefits.

3 Baby Food Diet

The idea with this 2007 diet was that you replace regular meals with 14 jars of baby food (between 20 and 100 calories each) throughout the day, and eat a low-calorie dinner. You might lose weight short-term, but once you start eating normally, chances are the weight will come back.

4 Cookie Diet

Founded by Dr. Sanford Siegal, eating cookies all day sounded like fun. Specially formulated weight-loss cookies would be consumed for breakfast, lunch and snacks for a total of nine cookies daily (60 calories each). While it recommended a healthy dinner for a calorie count around 1,200 daily, eating cookies all day isn't sustainable over the long haul.

5 Clay Diet

This one got some buzz a few years ago among celebs looking to drop pounds fast and "detox." But a diet consisting of clay powder stirred into water isn't just gross—it can be downright dangerous for your gut.

6 Five-Bite Diet

Created by obesity doctor Alwin Lewis, M.D., in 2007, you can eat whatever you choose to for lunch and dinner—no breakfast—but you only eat five bites of it, tops. The issue here is still severe caloric restriction.

7 Master Cleanse

Stretching back to the 1940s, when Stanley Burroughs launched the body-detox plan that involves drinking six-plus cups of a lemon juice, water, maple syrup and cayenne pepper mixture daily for anywhere from four to 14 days, the diet hit peak popularity when Beyoncé told an *Oprah* audience in 2007 that she lost 20 pounds in two weeks on it while preparing for a film role. Since then, its popularity has waned.

8 Fruitarian Diet

This diet made headlines after landing actor Ashton Kutcher in the hospital with an out-of-whack pancreas after he ate only fruit for one full month while preparing for the film role of Steve Jobs, who himself was a fruitarian. While dining on a variety of antioxidant-packed fruit sounds healthy, this diet, like most fad diets, is extremely restrictive. For most on it, 75 percent or more of what they eat daily is raw fruit. Depending on the person, they may nosh on nuts, seeds, beans or raw veggies.

21 Ways to Lose a Pound a Week

*Here are research-proven tips to help you cut calories,
burn more fat and shed weight for good.*

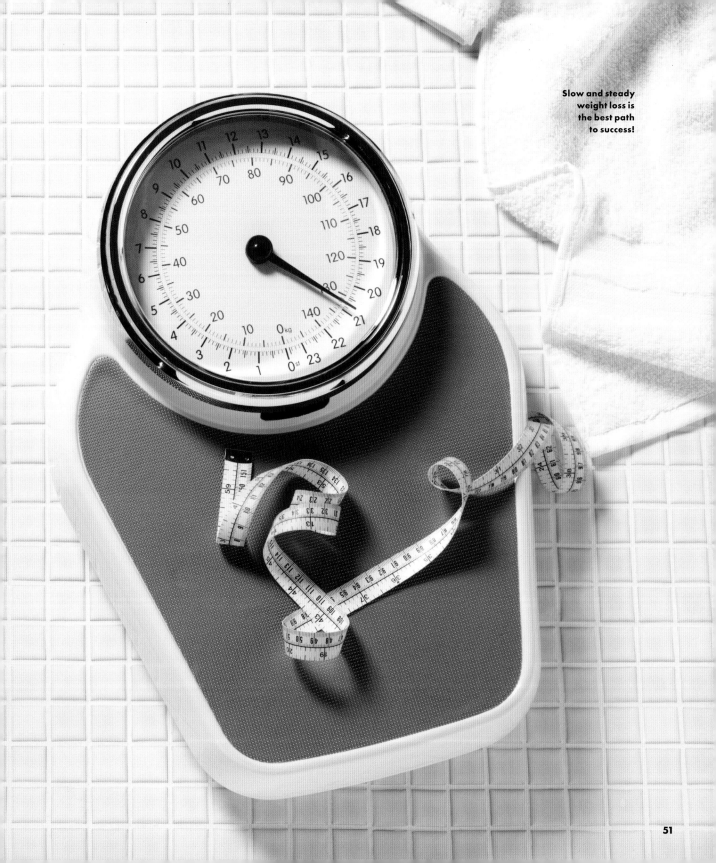

Slow and steady
weight loss is
the best path
to success!

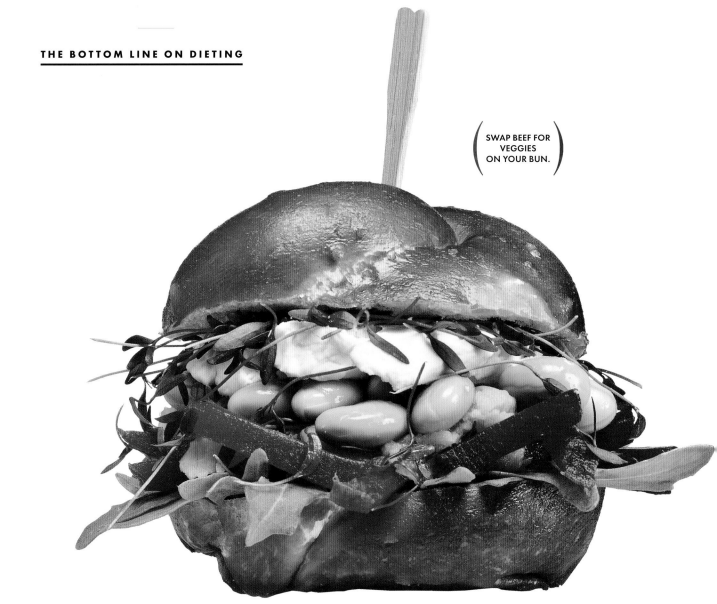

SWAP BEEF FOR
VEGGIES
ON YOUR BUN.

While many of us may desire a weight-loss solution that will help us shed 5 or more pounds per week, that's not a safe and sustainable rate of weight loss. Most health and nutrition experts recommend setting weight loss goals of 1 to 2 pounds a week for an attainable measure that will be more likely to stick over the long haul.

In order to lose 1 pound a week, you need to create a weekly deficit of 3,500 calories (that's the number of calories in a pound). That can be done by cutting back on portions, making lower-calorie swaps, or increasing the amount of exercise you do to burn off more calories.

Here, we'll walk you through 21 ways to drop a pound a week. Some will help you cut a few hundred calories, while others will trim 250 or fewer and should be combined with exercise to help you create a 500-calorie daily deficit. Combine a few if you'd like, or tackle one a week and add on once you've got the hang of it.

1 **Walk an Extra Hour Per Day** A 155-pound woman walking at a 17-minute mile (3.5 mph) pace could burn about 267 calories walking on a flat surface. Break that up into 20 minutes in the morning, 20 minutes during your lunch break and 20 minutes after dinner.

2 **Have a Meatless Burger** Save calories by enjoying a grilled portobello mushroom (about 22 calories) or a Boca All-American Classic Veggie Burger (90 calories) or similar veggie burger, instead of a 6-ounce 80/20 beef patty (425 calories).

3 **Trade a 20-Ounce Soda for Water** You know that soda isn't good for your health because it's packed with sugar and empty calories. If you swap a 20-ounce bottle of soda for seltzer water or a glass of water, you'd save 240 calories—not to mention at least 64 grams of sugar. This one daily change could result in 25 pounds gone in a year.

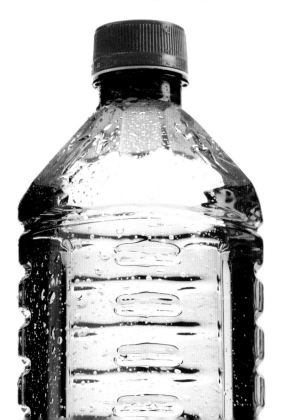

4 **Turn Off the TV** Many studies show an association between the hours a person spends watching TV and their likelihood of consuming more calories. One study had participants halve their TV watching time and found they burned an extra 120 calories per day than the group that didn't change their five-hour daily TV habit. Excess TV time has also been associated with obesity and Type 2 diabetes.

5 **Swap a Fast-Food Muffin for an English Muffin** Trade in that Chocolate Chunk Muffin at Starbucks (440 calories) for a light Thomas' English Muffin at home (100 calories) with 1 tablespoon of peanut butter (100 calories) and save 240 calories.

6 **Doggie-Bag Your Meal** Sure, you've heard this tip before, but research shows that the average restaurant entrée is about 1,200 calories (more than double what you should be eating at one meal). Ask your server to place half of the entrée on your plate and put the rest in a to-go container so you won't be tempted to eat it. You could save about 600 calories!

7 **Sip Broth-Based Soup Before a Meal** Having a low-cal soup may help you cut down on calories in the rest of your meal. A Penn State University study found that subjects who had soup before a lunch entrée reduced their total calorie intake at lunch by 20 percent, compared to when they didn't sip soup. That can translate into 240 calories saved.

8 **Strap on an Activity Monitor** The jury is still out on just how accurately "calories burned" are reported with many fitness wearables, but researchers find that doing more everyday activities results in more calories torched all day. If you walk briskly for 30 minutes and incorporate activities adding up to 10,000 steps a day, you'll likely burn 400 to 500 calories daily, which could mean a pound lost each week.

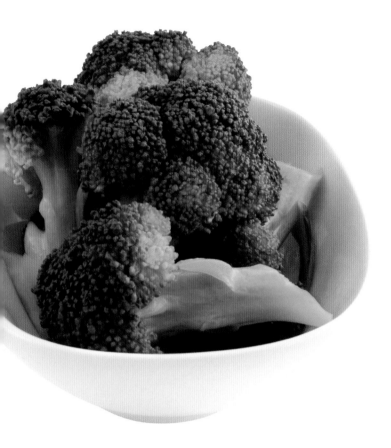

11 **Tackle Yard Chores** While this isn't something you'll probably do daily, incorporating gardening activities and yard work into your weekend will add up to major calories burned. The average calories burned for a 150-pound person doing these activities for an hour really rack up: mowing the lawn with a push mower (340); gardening and weeding (242); raking the lawn (272); heavy cleaning, like clearing out the garage or washing windows (238). Why not take advantage of a gorgeous day and torch calories while beautifying your property?

12 **Add Interval Training to Your Routine** Doing high-intensity interval training (HIIT) where you get your heart rate up for intervals throughout a workout can help you burn more fat, shed belly fat, and increase the afterburn effect, meaning you keep burning calories when you're done exercising. Choose an interval workout on the treadmill or elliptical; try a spinning class; or take a class at the gym incorporating these high-intensity spurts.

13 **Make an Effort to Fidget** Tapping your foot, wiggling in your chair and simply getting up more throughout the day can add up! You can burn 350 more calories in a day than someone who is more sedentary and still, according to studies.

9 **Choose Lower-Calorie Sides** When you're dining at a restaurant, swap French fries (with 273 calories for a cup) for one cup of steamed broccoli—hold the butter—and save about 230 calories.

10 **Prioritize Getting Seven to Eight Hours of Sleep** A recent meta-analysis of sleep studies found that partial sleep deprivation led to study participants consuming an extra 385 calories per day. Other studies discovered that shorting yourself on sleep can lead to hormonal changes that lead to overeating, a sluggish metabolism, higher insulin resistance levels, and a higher BMI. Get seven to eight hours of quality sleep per night to aid your weight-loss efforts.

14 **Leave Some Food on Your Plate** Eating one or two fewer bites at every meal could save about 150 calories a day, depending on what you're eating and how many meals you consume. That could add up to 15 pounds shaved off your frame in a year.

15 **Eat a Larger Breakfast** A Tel Aviv University study found that those who ate a larger meal in the morning lost 2.5 times more weight—and waistline circumference—than those who consumed the same amount of calories but had a larger dinner.

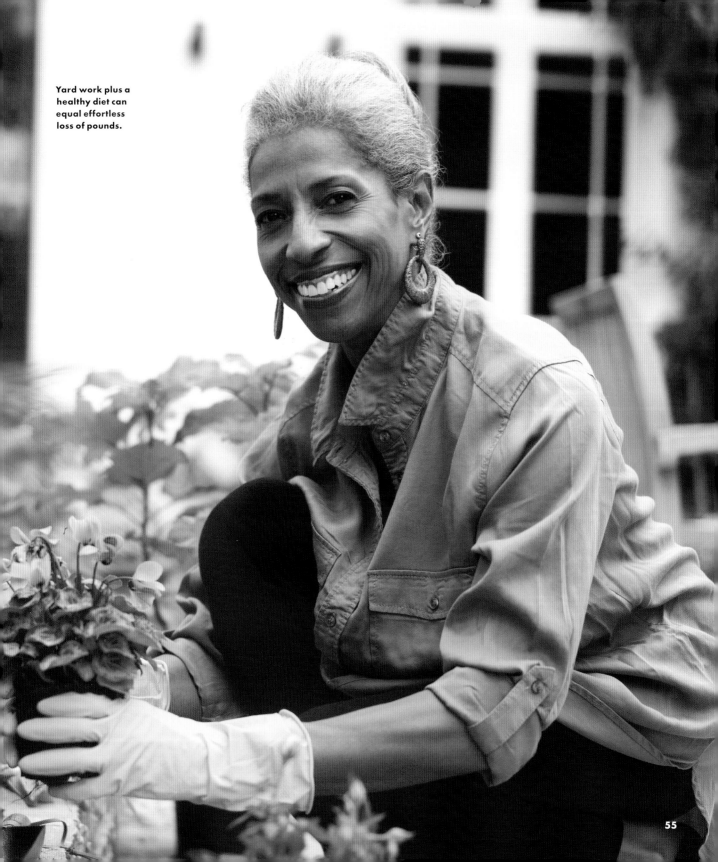

Yard work plus a
healthy diet can
equal effortless
loss of pounds.

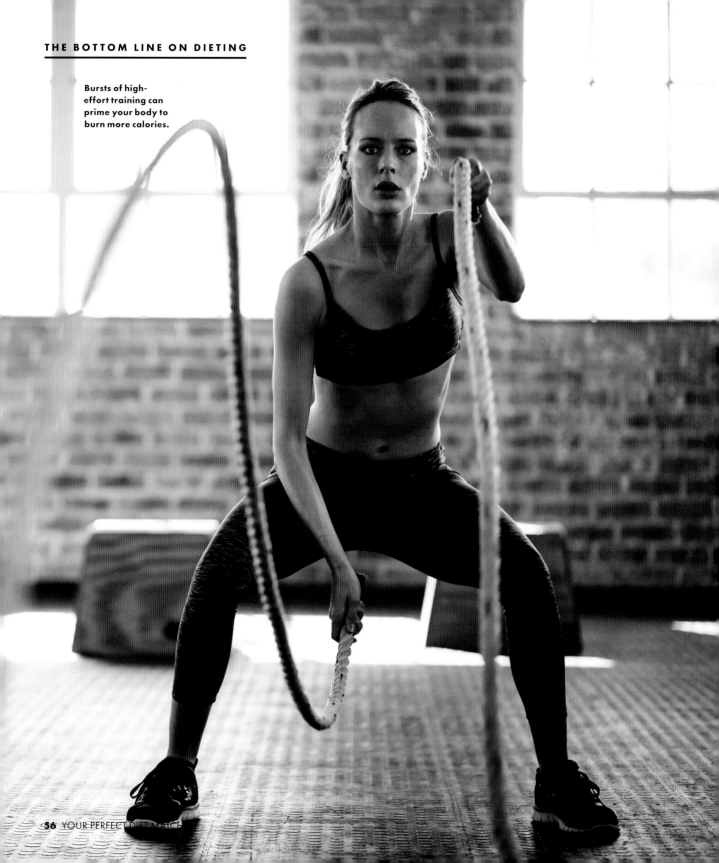

Bursts of high-effort training can prime your body to burn more calories.

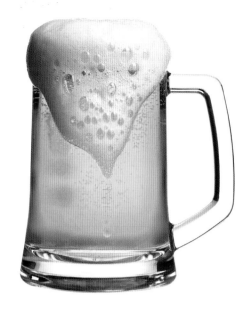

16 **Add Strength Training** Incorporating weight training into your fitness routine will help you burn more calories at rest. One study found that after inactive adults followed a resistance-training routine for 10 weeks, they increased resting metabolic rate (how many calories your body burns simply functioning) by 7 percent. More muscle mass can help you burn calories while sitting at your desk or napping by the pool.

17 **Cut Carbs in Half** Practicing portion control is an effective weight-loss strategy. Eat half a bagel (saving about 130 calories), use one slice of bread for your sandwich (saving about 120 calories), and keep rice or pasta to half-cup servings.

18 **Dine on Smaller Plates** Using smaller plates at mealtime can help curtail the amount of food you're eating. Halving the plate size led to a 30 percent reduction in the amount of food consumed on average in studies. Trading your 12-inch dinner plate for a salad plate will make a meal look larger, and you might save about 200 calories by eating less.

19 **Save Alcohol Consumption for the Weekends** Calories from alcohol count for 5 percent of adults' caloric intake, according to a study. The U.S. adult population consumes an average of almost 100 calories per day from alcoholic beverages. Keep it to the weekends for major calorie cutting.

20 **Chug More Water** Not only will it help fill you up, but it could also help you lose weight. In a study of middle-aged subjects who drank 17 ounces of water before their meal, they were found to consume fewer calories than members of the control group—and they lost about 4.5 pounds more after 12 weeks.

21 **Practice Mindful Eating Techniques** When was the last time you ate without distractions? When you turn off the TV, put away your phone and concentrate on the flavors, textures and smells of your dish, you might consume less food, studies show. That's because you're slowing your eating and it takes your brain 20 minutes to register that your stomach is full. Learning mindfulness techniques, like meditation and cognitive therapy, had a 97 percent impact on the weight loss of obese individuals in another study.

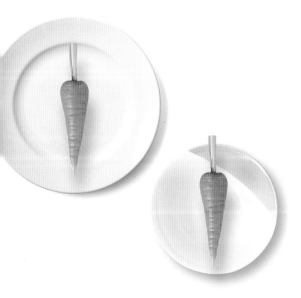

WHAT'S SABOTAGING YOUR SUCCESS?

All of us have different issues when it comes to food, fitness and habits. Take this quiz to pinpoint your struggles.

1. Which of these reasons resonates most for why you want to lose weight?

A. My doctor suggested it.

B. I want to look better for a specific event.

C. I want to have more energy, sleep better and feel healthier.

D. I want to lose weight because a family member suggested it.

E. I want to learn how to make better food choices.

2. The food struggle most challenging for me is:

A. Portion sizes—I tend to overeat.

B. I'm a foodie and love spending time with friends and family at restaurants.

C. I tend to reach for food when I'm stressed, bored or anxious.

D. Eating food off my kids' plates or eating too quickly around others.

E. I fall prey to eating junk food, fast food and sweets.

3. What do you find yourself doing after a long, tough day?

A. Lying on the couch with the remote, watching TV and dozing off.

B. Meeting up with friends or a partner for happy hour.

C. Eating a microwavable frozen dinner or takeout meal, paired with a strong drink, to help me unwind after a long day at the office.

D. Cleaning up after the family dinner, prepping for the next day and, finally, relaxing with my partner.

E. Eating pizza, chips or ice cream on my couch.

4. How do you feel about most weight-loss plans?

A. They are too restrictive and leave me feeling hungry.

B. They limit my ability to live my life and dine out.

C. They are way too complicated, expensive and time-consuming.

D. They involve buying special foods, requiring me to make two dinners for my family, and I feel isolated when I get stuck.

E. They require eating bland or expensive foods, and I can't wait to lose and be done.

5. What kind of diet plan sounds most appealing?

A. One that my doctor prescribes, with a list of foods I can and cannot eat.

B. A diet that allows me the flexibility to go out or be able to enjoy myself at parties.

C. One that's simple, doesn't involve meal prep and cooking, where I'm told what to eat—and maybe it comes delivered to my front door.

D. A plan where there's a robust online community or some in-person support and accountability.

E. A healthy-eating plan that is easy to stick to; provides flexibility; and involves whole, natural foods—without counting and calculating.

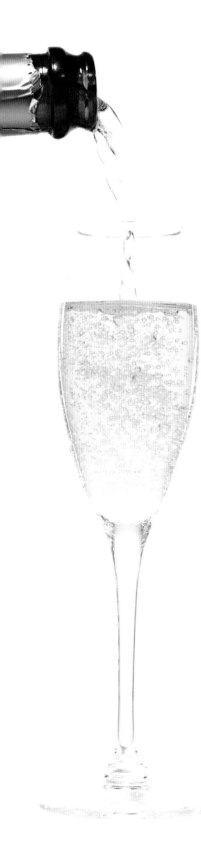

Answers

Tally up your answers and learn what's holding you back.

MOSTLY A's

• Your "Why" Needs to Change

You know it's important to get to a healthy weight in order to improve your overall health and well-being as well as reduce your risk for certain diseases. If a poor diagnosis at the physician's office isn't enough to motivate you, consider the benefits of weight loss—like being able to play with your children, getting better sleep or having more energy. A weight-loss plan that addresses a health issue, like hypertension (DASH) or heart disease (South Beach Diet) might be a good fit. You may also find it beneficial to work with a nutritionist to address your specific health needs.

MOSTLY B's

• Your Social Calendar

You love to eat out and celebrate with friends or entertain at home. Trouble is, restaurant meals tend to have tons more calories and fat than meals made at home. Limit your dining out to two nights a week—and keep an eye on food portions and alcohol intake, since those might interfere with your best intentions. Look for a plan that has flexibility, like WW, Noom or The Dubrow Diet, so you don't have to sacrifice your social life.

MOSTLY C's

• Your Stress-Filled Life

You have a lot on your plate—and we're not talking food. With your jam-packed work schedule and personal life, you need to find healthy ways to handle stress in order to stick to your plan. Consider meditation, daily exercise…even finding a few moments of down time to relax with loved ones. You would benefit from a diet plan that makes food selection easy. Try one that delivers food to your doorstep, like the South Beach Diet. You also might like an intermittent-fasting plan so you don't have to think about prepping all your meals—just eat during the specified time window!

MOSTLY D's

• You're Doing This Alone

You've probably found that past diets didn't work when you were going it alone, buying foods the rest of the family wouldn't eat and eating boring salads when out to dinner with loved ones. You'll benefit by enlisting your family to help you stick to your weight-loss intentions, hold you accountable and not give you grief when you're ditching unhealthy foods. Ultimately, this has to be something you are ready to do and can get help with to make it last. A diet with a robust community—like Noom or WW—where you can get support from like-minded people could help you find the encouragement you need.

MOSTLY E's

• You're Eating the Wrong Foods

You know what you should be eating (e.g., grilled chicken instead of fried), but ultimately, you need some guidance in making healthier food choices that will help you feel good and lose weight. Try a plan like Whole30 or Paleo, where you'll eliminate processed foods and get reacquainted with good-for-you, wholesome foods. You may even find you like eating healthy!

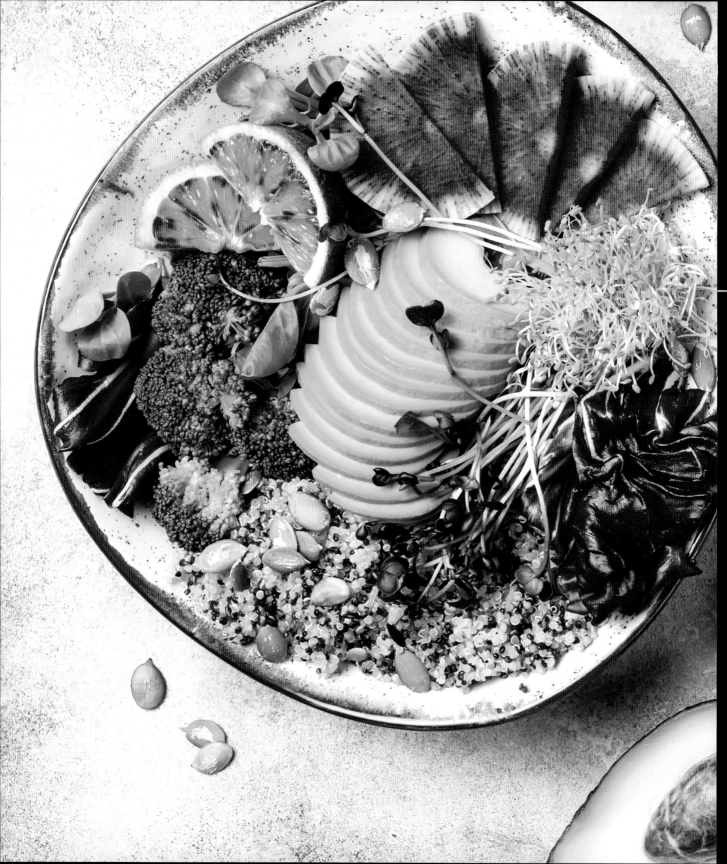

Chapter 2

FIND THE RIGHT PLAN

FIND THE RIGHT PLAN

Finding the foods that are best for your body isn't as hard as it sounds.

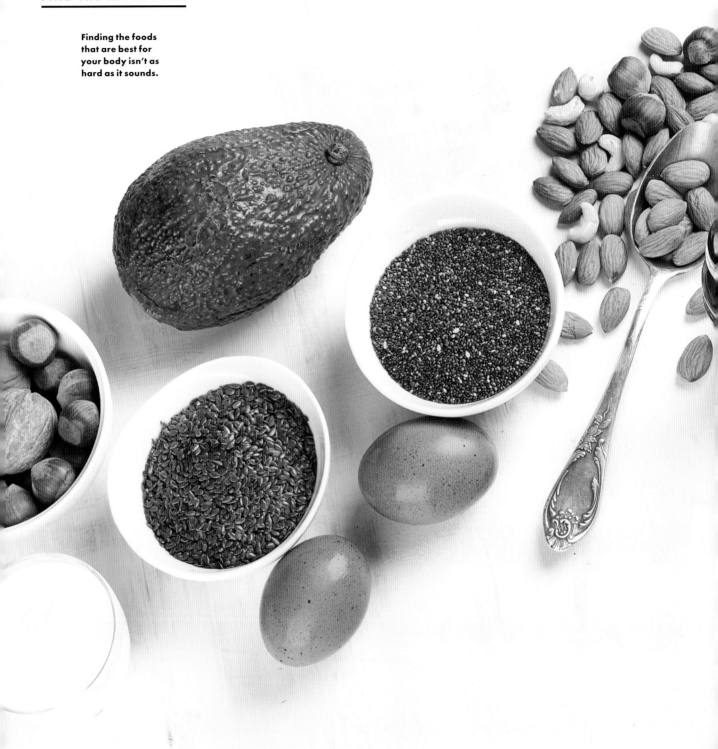

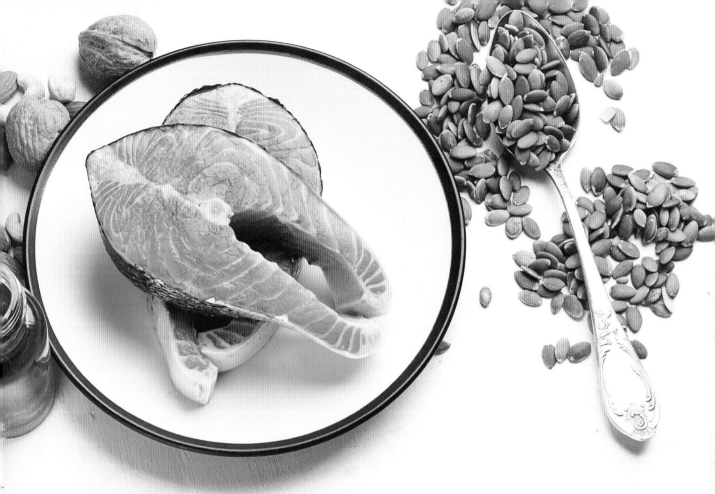

Plan for Your Health

When it comes to your well-being, how and what you eat can make all the difference in helping you feel better.

Diet. The word itself can make you feel like you're on a mission. But once the initial motivation wears off, it can be tough to stick to any food plan. That's why it's so important to tailor a diet to specific health goals. "If a plan doesn't make you feel well, takes too much time, or isn't a fit for your lifestyle, it'll fizzle out fast," says Cynthia Sass, M.P.H., R.D., a New York City and Los Angeles-based private-practice nutritionist. "The only plans that work are those you can stick with. If you know in your gut that you can't see yourself continuing a plan six weeks or six months down the road, it's not right for you."

Even if you feel a diet is doable over the long haul, another crucial element is ensuring it's what your body needs. To see success, target your diet to a specific goal, such as the ones below.

If You Want to Lower Blood Sugar

The right diet can do wonders for regulating blood sugar levels. "Sometimes you can be eating within the calorie range, but having the wrong foods," says Katrina Haghighi, R.D.N., a nutritionist at Smart Dimensions MemorialCare Surgical Weight Loss Center at Orange Coast Medical Center in Fountain Valley, California. "Not every calorie is created equal."

Too much sugar will keep insulin levels high and your body in fat-storage mode, so load up on whole foods and vegetables—but try to avoid eating more than two servings of fruit a day when you're looking to lose weight. Pair fruit with a protein to slow the absorption of sugar into the bloodstream and avoid insulin spikes. "The more processed food is, the more rapidly it's absorbed into the bloodstream, causing insulin peaks," Haghighi says. "Sometimes the sugar is so high that when levels start to go back to normal, the blood sugar level goes a bit below and signals the brain to crave *more* sugar."

Beware of added sugars. It's best to have sweeteners in the most natural form possible, so skip OJ in favor of eating an orange. "Even if you squeeze orange juice at home, there's hardly any fiber it in," Haghighi says. "It'll cause a rush of sugar going into your bloodstream. But if you eat an orange, the brain gets the message that you are chewing, taking longer for you to eat it—plus, you're getting fiber from the fruit itself."

To regulate blood sugar, spread carbohydrates throughout the day so there's an even flow, and stick with whole foods that aren't processed in a factory. Even prepackaged or microwavable foods that claim to be healthy typically aren't. "I tell my patients to read the ingredient list because [health claims on labels] are essentially lying," Haghighi says. "[Manufacturing companies] can change words around or use a word you don't know that stands for another ingredient." For example, if the label claims to be whole-wheat bread, make sure it has whole-wheat flour—if it says enriched or bleached, then it's not as healthy as it claims to be. Whole-grain foods keep you full longer. Load up on low-glycemic foods, proteins and healthy fats.

Another option to lower blood sugar is to follow the Mediterranean diet, which features plenty of vegetables, a moderate amount of protein and a low amount of carbs, plus an emphasis on healthy fats, such as olive oil. Research has shown that subjects on a Mediterranean diet had better control over blood sugar levels, as well as improved heart health. Another study found those on a Mediterranean diet who got at least 30 percent of their calories from fat (mostly from olive oil) were better able to manage their diabetes symptoms without needing medication, compared to those on a lower-fat diet.

There's also evidence that the ketogenic diet, which is 70 percent fat, 20 percent protein and 10 percent carbs, may help lower and stabilize blood sugar levels, says Robert Silverman, D.C., M.S., C.N.S. By slashing carbs, you'll naturally reduce sugar from your diet, he explains.

If You Want to Reverse Diabetes

When people adjust their diet to eat healthier and lose weight, they can often lower their dosage

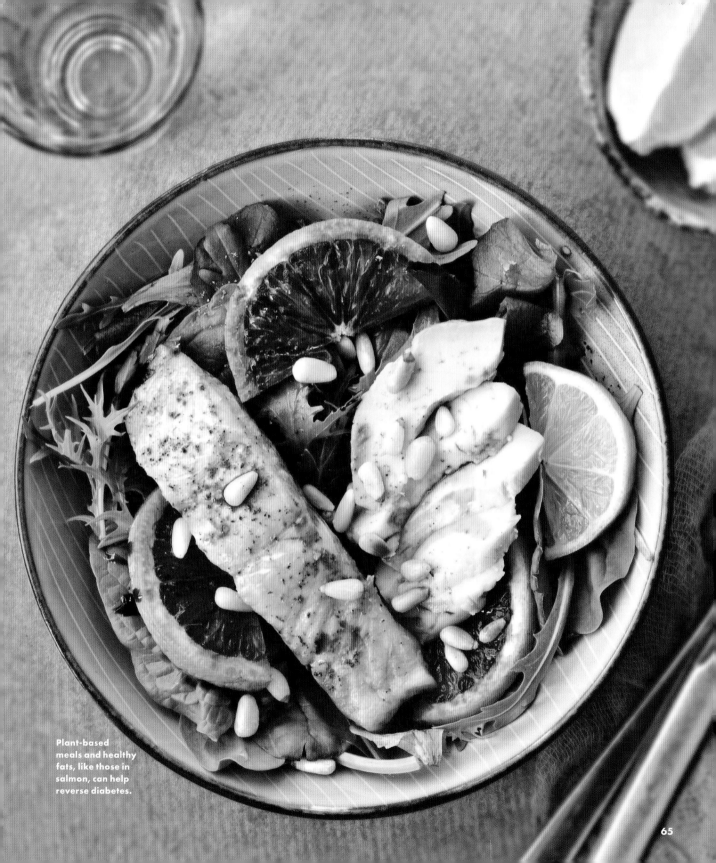

Plant-based meals and healthy fats, like those in salmon, can help reverse diabetes.

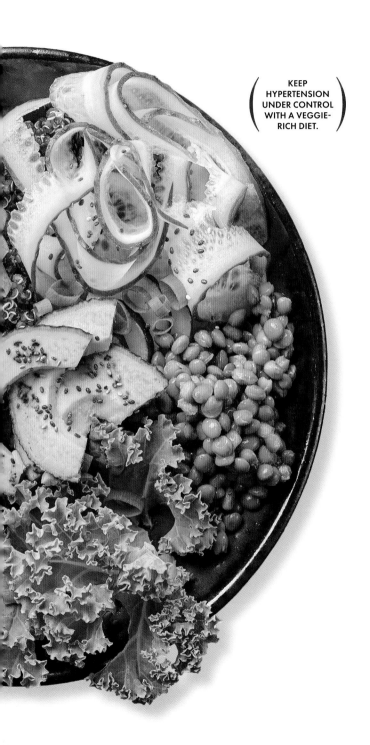

KEEP HYPERTENSION UNDER CONTROL WITH A VEGGIE-RICH DIET.

of diabetes and blood pressure medications. "People always think it's the medications that can reverse diabetes, but those just help alleviate the symptoms—they don't cure the actual disease," Haghighi says. "A 5 percent to 10 percent weight loss can change that."

Look for a plan similar to those that will help manage blood sugar levels and stay within your calorie range. "Stick to a diet high in nonstarchy vegetables, moderate in protein, with mostly monounsaturated fat, and is moderate in carbohydrates that are whole-food based, high fiber and appropriately timed," recommends Sass. "That means not eating the bulk of your carbs during one part of the day, like at night, and trying to eat slightly larger portions during more-active hours of the day and smaller portions around less-active times of the day." If your job tends to be sedentary, for example, and you know you won't be active or exercise in the a.m., avoid having a carb-heavy breakfast, she says. "But if you take a walk after lunch, you can include some healthy carbs in your lunch meal."

If You Want to Lower Cholesterol

A flexitarian diet—which involves slashing meat intake and prioritizing veggie-packed dishes, while avoiding sweets and processed foods—is the way to go, says Silverman. Loading up on plant-based meals naturally lowers cholesterol. "The American Medical Association said that being semi-vegetarian is nutritionally sound as long as you include the essential nutrients," Silverman says. "Any diet that's low in sugar is good, because sugar leads to high triglycerides, which leads to high cholesterol."

When you're eating to lower bad cholesterol, avoiding trans fats is key, but you'll also want to eat foods that raise good cholesterol, by adding healthy fats like olive or coconut oil. Fatty fish with omega-3s can reduce triglycerides. And chow down on soluble fiber, which is found in nuts, seeds, beans, lentils, oat bran, barley and some fruits and vegetables.

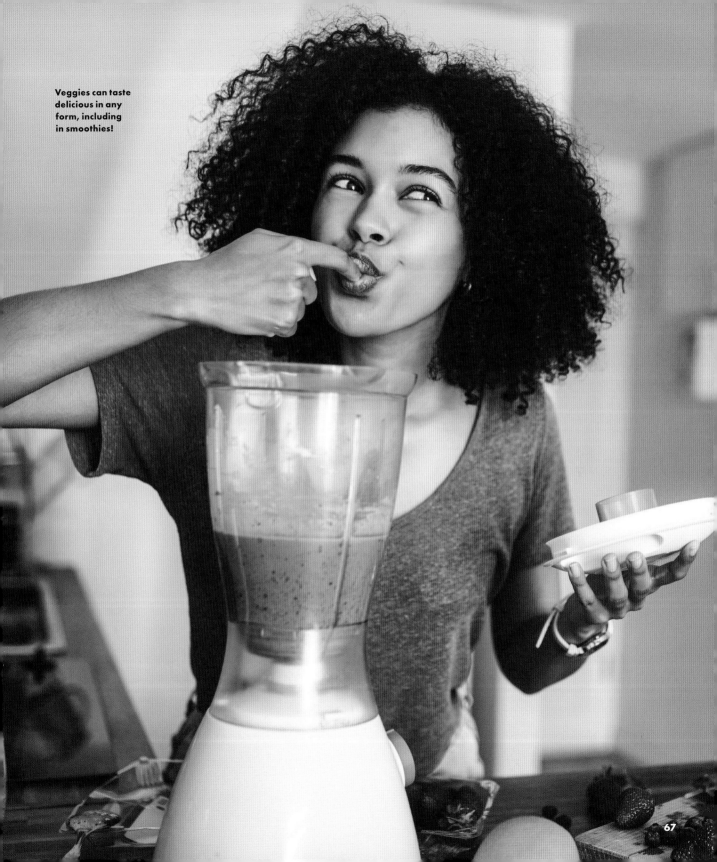

Veggies can taste delicious in any form, including in smoothies!

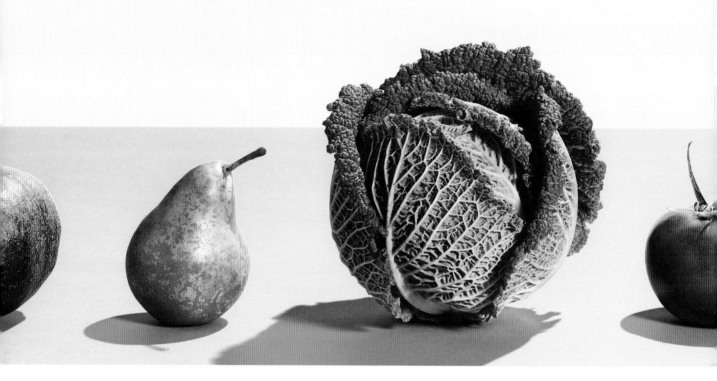

If You Want to Control Salt Intake

This is exactly what the DASH diet—which stands for Dietary Approaches to Stop Hypertension—is for, and numerous studies have proven its efficacy. "It truly fights high blood pressure," says Silverman. "It's praised for its nutritional completeness and safety, as well as for its role in supporting heart health." DASH emphasizes fruits, vegetables and low or nonfat dairy, and includes whole grains, nuts and beans, lean meats, poultry and fish. It's low in fat and high in fiber, and limits sodium. Another perk is that the DASH diet may lower your risk for depression, according to a recent study from Rush University Medical Center in Chicago.

"If you have hypertension, you should get no more than 1,500 mg of sodium a day, and the general population should limit it to 2,300 mg," says Haghighi. (For comparison: The average American eats an average of 3,400 mg of sodium per day, according to the FDA.) "I always tell patients to look at the sodium in any kind of packaged meal, and to check the portion sizes, since one small microwavable meal can contain two portion sizes, and when people eat the whole thing they go over their recommended sodium intake," Haghighi suggests. Instead, opt for fresh foods and use natural spices or salt-free seasonings. If you were eating a high-salt diet, it may take a while for your natural tastes to adjust.

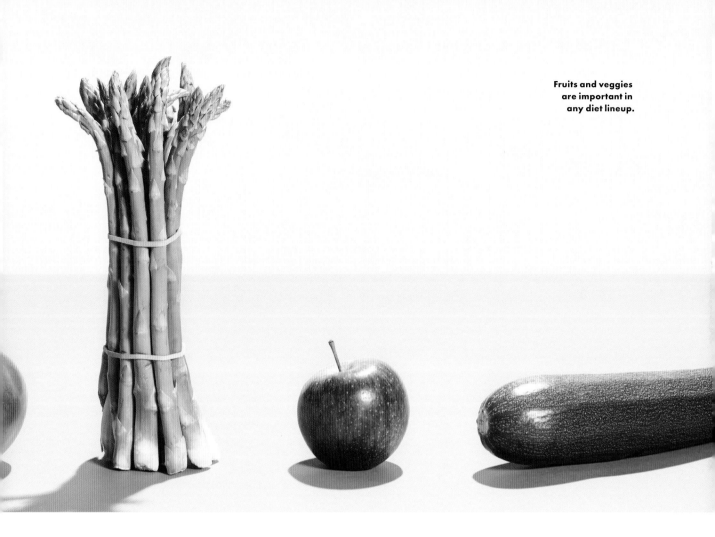

If You Want to Lose Weight

This may be the most common health concern for starting a diet, but "there is no one [diet example] to share here," Sass says. What's sustainable for you is the plan that will be best for losing weight and keeping it off long-term, she adds. "If you don't like to cook or don't have time to do so, a plan that requires lots of cooking and meal prep isn't going to work. Long-term weight loss is about developing a lifestyle, not going on and going off a diet," Sass says. No matter which you choose, it's all about watching your calories, and loading up on the right foods.

Managing portion sizes is crucial for success. "Invest in a food scale," says Haghighi. "When you keep weighing chicken, you'll see what 4 ounces really looks like." It's important to make healthy habits, like meal planning and prepping for the week, part of your lifestyle. "I always say, 'If I fail to plan, I plan to fail,'" says Haghighi. It's a lot easier to turn down the office birthday cake when you've packed a healthy snack to keep you on track.

The ketogenic diet is Silverman's go-to plan for lasting weight loss. "In America we think fat makes you fat, but keto can bring great changes in weight loss; the results are outstanding." Silverman believes it's sustainable as a lifestyle, so you won't put back on the pounds as long as you stick with it.

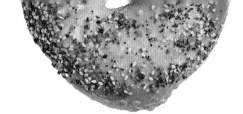

WHICH WEIGHT-LOSS PROGRAM IS BEST FOR YOU?

*Not every meal plan is created equal.
This quiz can help you determine which diet best suits your style.*

1. How much do you like to cook?

    A. I'm basically Julia Child.

    B. I'm not ready for *Chopped*, but I know the basics.

    C. Does microwaving count?

Many times, when people start a diet, they're often surprised at how much time they require—not only with cooking, but with shopping and prepping the ingredients. While you can get by with less cooking on plans like intuitive eating, Mediterranean, WW and flexitarian, keto, Paleo and some other low-carb plans are notorious for being high maintenance. But thankfully, meal delivery—available for many different eating styles —can be a lifesaver for the culinarily challenged.

2. What's your favorite source of protein? Check all that apply.

    ☐ Meat and poultry

    ☐ Fish

    ☐ Beans

    ☐ Dairy

    ☐ Tofu

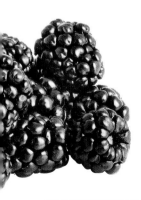

This is actually one of the key questions to ask yourself when choosing a plan: While almost every diet emphasizes vegetables, protein sources vary widely. Carnivores may want to consider one of the low-carb (Atkins, Paleo, keto, bone broth, South Beach) or high-fat (keto) plans; you can also eat fish on all these diets.

If you like seafood but not meat, try the Mediterranean, DASH or MIND diets. For bean and tofu lovers, there are the DASH, MIND, Mediterranean, vegan/ vegetarian and F-Factor programs. Love your milk and cheese? Try WW, Setpoint, carb cycling, vegetarian or flexitarian (and you can eat cheese, but not milk, on keto).

3. When you think about a life without bread, what's your reaction?

    A. I'd rather die.

    B. I'd miss it, but I could make do.

    C. The best invention of the 21st century were those sandwiches that replaced the bread with fried chicken.

Plans like DASH, MIND, Mediterranean, vegan/ vegetarian and F-Factor allow pasta and bread (ideally the whole-grain, high-fiber versions). If you rarely crave these, any of the low-carb diets can be a good fit.

4. When was the last time you skipped a meal?

    A. 1994

    B. Last month

    C. This morning

If you're not married to the three-meals-a-day concept, intermittent fasting might be for you. Try The Fast Diet or The Dubrow Diet.

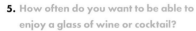

5. How often do you want to be able to
enjoy a glass of wine or cocktail?

   A. Every darn day!

   B. A couple of times a week, on weekends.

   C. I don't drink.

While some diets (Whole30, juicing) forbid alcohol,
moderate alcohol consumption is allowed on the
Mediterranean, intuitive eating and WW plans;
keto and Paleo allow grain-free spirits.

6. How would you rank your nutritional
knowledge?

   A. I could be a dietitian.

   B. I'm in the middle.

   C. I know Twinkies aren't healthy, but that's about it.

Diets like Paleo, keto and Whole30 have simple rules:
You stop eating ABC foods and start enjoying XYZ foods.
If you're not a nutrition whiz, one of these easy-to-follow
diets may be a good fit for you.

7. How would you describe your
relationship with vegetables?

   A. We're madly in love.

   B. I don't mind them…as a friend.

   C. We're frenemies. I just barely tolerate them.

While most plans emphasize eating loads of vegetables,
keto does limit them somewhat. Diets like juicing help
disguise them in smoothies.

8. What are the chances of you using a food scale?

   A. No problem! I'm basically a frustrated scientist.

   B. I'd find it a bit annoying, but could deal.

   C. When hell freezes over.

Some diets—like WW—are all about portion control,
which means lots of measuring. If this brings back bad
memories of high school science, a more free-range plan
may be a better fit.

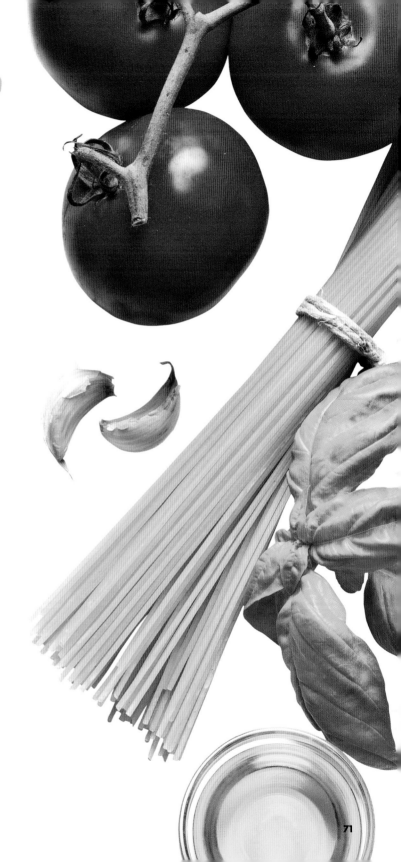

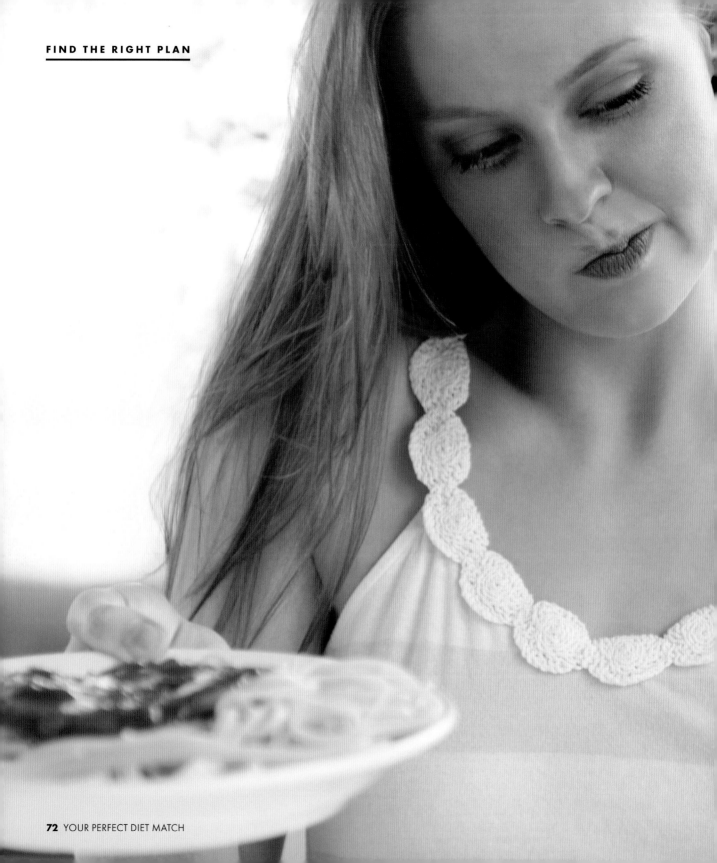

How 28 Different Diets Stack Up

Before you read detailed descriptions of the diets on the following pages, see how they compare to one another based on their nutrition, the foods you'll have to avoid, the expense of following each one and the amount of work it'll require to stick to the program.

Find out what you'll really be eating before committing to a diet program.

FIND THE RIGHT PLAN

	ALLOWS FRUIT	ALLOWS DAIRY	ALLOWS ALCOHOL	CONSIDERED LOW-CARB	
THE 5-FACTOR DIET	●	●	●		
ALKALINE DIET	●	●	●		
ATKINS DIET (Including later phases)	●	●	●	●	
BONE BROTH DIET	●	●		●	
CARB CYCLING DIET	●	●	●	●	
THE DASH DIET	●	●	●		
DR. GUNDRY'S DIET EVOLUTION	●	●	●		
THE DUBROW DIET	●	●	●	●	
THE F-FACTOR DIET	●	●	●		
THE FLEXITARIAN DIET	●	●	●		
INTERMITTENT FASTING DIET	●	●	●		
INTUITIVE EATING DIET	●	●	●		
JUICING DIET	●				
THE KETO DIET	●	●	●	●	

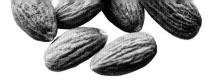

	VEGETARIAN-FRIENDLY	ENCOURAGES EXERCISE/ HAS FITNESS COMPONENT	EXPENSIVE $-$$$$*	DIFFICULTY TO FOLLOW ON 1 TO 10 SCALE**
	●	●	$$	3
	●		$$$	7
	●		$$	4
			$$	8
	●		$	9
	●	●	$$	4
	●		$	5
	●		$	5
	●		$$	3
	●		$$	4
	●	●	$	6
	●	●	$	2
	●		$$$	6
			$$$	8

*calls for organic or high-priced ingredients, like grass-fed meat
**1 = meals are easy to assemble and eat on the go;
   10 = lots of restrictions and requires more meal prep

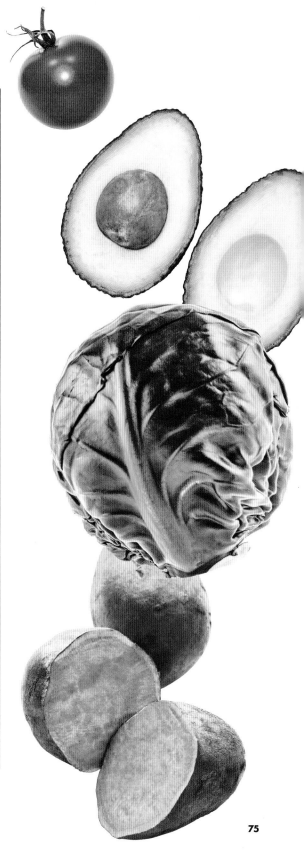

	ALLOWS FRUIT	ALLOWS DAIRY	ALLOWS ALCOHOL	CONSIDERED LOW-CARB	
THE LOSE YOUR BELLY DIET	●	●			
MEDITERRANEAN DIET	●	●	●		
THE MIND DIET	●	●	●		
NOOM	●	●	●		
THE PALEO DIET	●		●	●	
THE PLANT PARADOX DIET	●	●			
PORTION CONTROL DIET	●	●	●		
RAW FOOD DIET	●				
THE SETPOINT DIET	●	●	●	●	
THE SOUTH BEACH DIET	●	●	●	●	
THERAPEUTIC LIFESTYLE CHANGES DIET	●	●	●		
VEGAN/ VEGETARIAN/ PLANT-BASED DIETS	●		●		
THE WHOLE30 PROGRAM	●				
WW	●	●	●		

	VEGETARIAN-FRIENDLY	ENCOURAGES EXERCISE/ HAS FITNESS COMPONENT	EXPENSIVE $-$$$$*	DIFFICULTY TO FOLLOW ON 1 TO 10 SCALE**
	○	●	$$$$	8
	○	●	$	3
	○		$	3
	○	●	$$$	4
	○	●	$$$	7
	○		$	2
	○		$	1
	○		$$	9
	○	●	$	3
	○	●	$$	6
	○	●	$	2
	○		$$	8
	○		$$$	8
	○	●	$$	2

*calls for organic or high-priced ingredients, like grass-fed meat
** 1 = meals are easy to assemble and eat on the go;
   10 = lots of restrictions and requires more meal prep

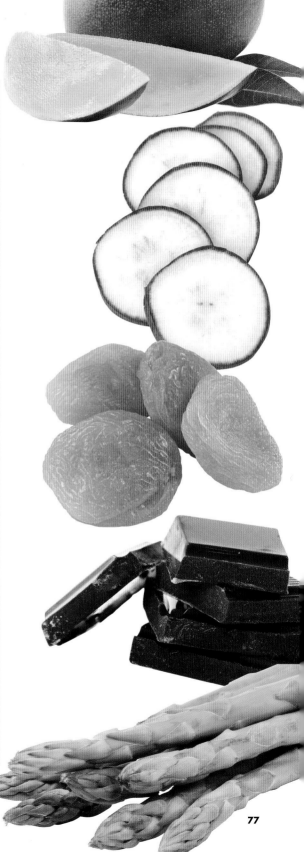

The 5-Factor Diet

Want to lose weight and work out like you hired a celebrity trainer to help you? You might find success with this weight-loss plan.

What Is It?

Celebrity fitness trainer Harley Pasternak created The 5-Factor Diet in 2005 when he published a book with the same name. Known for shaping Hollywood's hottest bodies, including Katy Perry, Kanye West, Lady Gaga and many more, Pasternak decided to dip his toes into a nutrition and lifestyle program for the masses with this plan.

The concept is simple: Eat five meals a day with five core ingredients in each recipe (that can be ready in five minutes or less) and complete five, 25-minute workouts a week (consisting of five, 5-minute segments) for weight-loss success in five weeks.

How It Works

By eating the five foods in the plan for five meals daily (breakfast, lunch, dinner and two snacks) you'll keep blood sugar levels stable so you're less likely to overeat. No calorie counting required. Pasternak also says that eating this way will give you more energy, ignite metabolism, improve mood and reduce stress.

"Overall, this seems like a pretty healthy lifestyle plan, emphasizing the importance of eating protein and fiber, both of which are satiating, as well as smaller meals and an overall well-balanced diet," says Amy Gorin, M.S., R.D.N., owner of Amy Gorin Nutrition in the New York City area. "It also encourages limiting many processed foods and high-calorie drinks, both of which should help with weight loss."

There's even a cheat day built into the plan so you can enjoy your favorite foods and indulge during special-occasion meals. Fitness is a big component of this plan— particularly strength training.

What You'll Eat

The five foods you'll eat in each meal include a lean protein (chicken breast, egg whites, fish, cottage cheese); a complex carb (apples, broccoli, strawberries, lettuce); foods with 5 to 10 grams of fiber (beans, whole-grain cereal, no-flour wheat breads); a "good" fat (fish oil, olive oil); and a sugar-free drink. Pasternak pushes lower-GI foods like steel-cut oatmeal, berries, sweet potatoes and lentils.

Foods to Avoid

You can eat whatever you want on your cheat day, so you don't have to avoid any items. Still, Pasternak suggests limiting "bad fats," including saturated fats (whole milk, butter, egg yolks, coconut oil) and trans fats (found in some processed foods).

THE PROS

- Fitness plays a key part: The workouts have five, 5-minute exercises to do five days each week.

- Eating low-GI foods can help keep blood sugar levels low after eating.

- If you hate meal prep, you may like the quick, easy-to-prepare recipes this plan outlines. You can find wholesome options that fit into this plan.

THE CONS

- If you can't make time to eat every few hours, this diet could be a challenge.

- Frequent restaurant diners might struggle with learning how to navigate menus on the diet, although you can find options.

- "I have concerns that the plan doesn't address different calorie needs of individuals," says Gorin. "These needs vary based on factors like age, gender and exercise habits."

- Over the long term, The 5-Factor Diet may be difficult to follow as life gets in the way, says Gorin. "You may have a wedding and a birthday fall in the same week. So then which do you choose for your cheat day?"

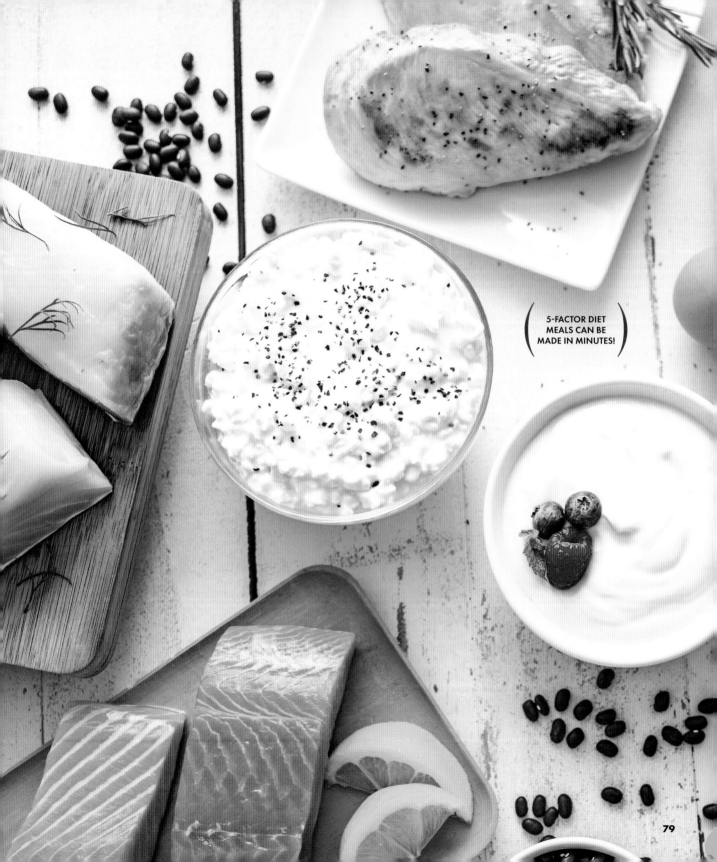

5-FACTOR DIET
MEALS CAN BE
MADE IN MINUTES!

Alkaline Diet

This plant-based (and celebrity-endorsed) program is designed to help reduce inflammation in the body.

What Is It?

"The premise of this diet is that you eat foods that slightly increase the pH of the urine" [not the blood, which your body carefully regulates], says Sonya Angelone, M.S., R.D.N., a spokesperson for the Academy of Nutrition and Dietetics.

Proponents of this plan believe that achieving an alkaline pH will help your body burn fat so you ultimately lose weight. They also maintain that it helps promote optimal energy (so you won't be too tired to work out) and proper body functioning. Celebrity fans have included Kelly Ripa, Gisele Bündchen and Victoria Beckham.

How It Works

This plan is based on the acid-alkaline theory of disease: Certain foods, when processed in the body, leave behind something called acidic ash, which can increase inflammation, explains Jennifer Koslo, R.D.N. Since obesity is a state of low-grade systemic inflammation, the theory is that by reducing this inflammation you can then spur weight loss. Other benefits may include preserving muscle mass, increasing bone density, improving cognitive function and reducing the risk of hypertension.

What You'll Eat

Eighty percent of what you eat will be alkaline-forming foods; 20 percent (or less) will be non-alkaline-forming foods. Alkaline foods are those that are low in sugar; high in water content; contain minerals such as magnesium, potassium, calcium and phosphorus; and have a negative or low PRAL score. The PRAL—the potential renal acid load—of a food measures its acid excretion in the urine, says Angelone. That means that veggies like leafy greens, broccoli and Brussels sprouts are the mainstays of this diet. "Vegetables tend to promote alkalinity in the body," says Angelone.

In addition, you can eat low-sugar fruits like berries; raw seeds and nuts; healthy fats and oils; and plant-based proteins like lentils. You're also allowed a small amount of acid-forming foods; these include meats, dairy, seafood, eggs, sugar, alcohol and processed foods.

Foods to Avoid

No foods are completely banned, but many items you're used to eating—bread, cheese, yogurt, sweets and alcohol—are very limited. "The goal is to influence the body's response to a meal," says Angelone.

THE PROS

- This diet encourages the consumption of vegetables, which is the tried-and-true basis of most successful weight-loss plans.

- It significantly limits high-calorie processed foods and sugars, which are often associated with weight gain.

- It's a diet that's high in fiber, which helps you feel full longer and avoid blood sugar spikes that can lead to overeating.

THE CONS

- This restrictive and inflexible diet can be hard to stick to, and can leave you feeling deprived.

- Healthy, acid-forming foods aren't necessarily harmful and don't need to be avoided, says Sonya Angelone, R.D.N. They can be part of a healthy diet.

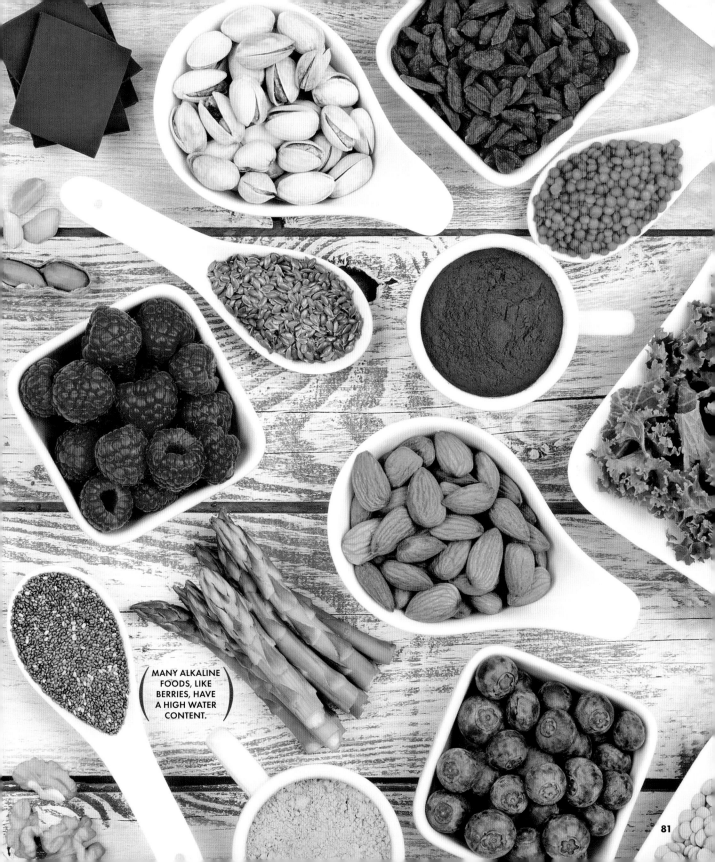

MANY ALKALINE FOODS, LIKE BERRIES, HAVE A HIGH WATER CONTENT.

Atkins Diet

This low-carb weight-loss plan will help you lose weight, but it might not be sustainable for everyone.

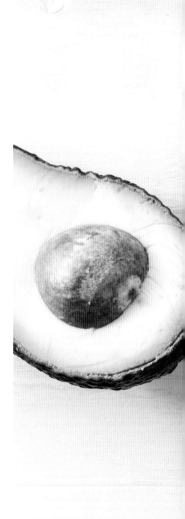

What Is It?

Yes, the weight-loss plan that has gone in and out of style is still alive and kicking nearly 50 years later.

Created by the late cardiologist Dr. Robert Atkins, the book *Dr. Atkins' Diet Revolution: The High-Calorie Way to Stay Thin Forever* was published in 1972 and claimed that you can lose weight by eating as much protein and fat as you want, as long as you avoid foods high in carbs. The book and diet have been updated over the years since it was published, and research has caught up with the plan—proving that a low-carb diet can help people lose weight.

But not everyone is a fan. "I've always been critical of the low-carb diets," says Los Angeles–based Mascha Davis, M.P.H., R.D.N., national media spokeswoman for the Academy of Nutrition and Dietetics. "Any time that you cut out a whole food group, people are going to lose weight, particularly when it's the food group that makes up the majority of your calories. Sure, it's effective in the short-term. Is it sustainable? Absolutely not," she adds.

How It Works

The original Atkins Diet has you following this plan: Phase 1 (20-25 daily net carbs for two weeks); Phase 2 (25-50 daily net carbs); Phase 3 (50-80 daily net carbs); Phase 4 (80-100 daily net carbs). Net carbs are calculated by taking the total carb content of the food (per serving) minus the fiber content. Thanks to technological advances, it's much easier to do this calculation using smartphone apps to research foods' nutritional content.

There's also an Atkins 40 Diet plan, based on portion control and eating 40 grams of net carbs per day. This plan is recommended if you have fewer than 40 pounds to lose, are breastfeeding, or want a wider variety of food choices to start out with.

What You'll Eat

This is the diet that had everyone eating more bacon in the '90s.

Although the first phase of Atkins is strict, the next few phases allow for gradual flexibility when it comes to adding a variety of foods in your diet. While Phase 4 —that's around 80 to 100 grams of carbs daily—is still considered low-carb, there's room in that plan for pasta or a slice of pizza.

You'll eat meat, full-fat dairy, nuts and seeds, peanut butter, avocados,

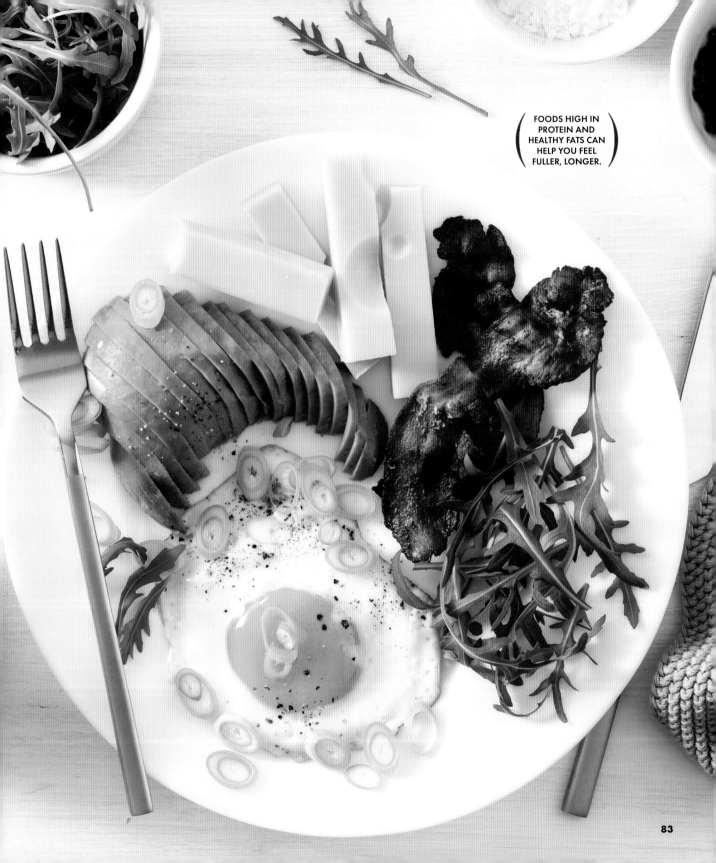

FOODS HIGH IN PROTEIN AND HEALTHY FATS CAN HELP YOU FEEL FULLER, LONGER.

fish and lots of low-carb veggies like green vegetables and tomatoes.

What to Avoid

In this early phase, you'll stay away from sugar, desserts, bagels, high-carb bread products, most grains, potatoes, high-carb vegetables (like carrots) and high-carb fruits (apples, bananas, grapes), as well as lentils.

According to the Atkins plan's website, drinking alcohol can slow your weight loss, since you'll be burning alcohol instead of fat. That being said, in a later phase of Atkins, or if you're following the Atkins 40 program, a glass of wine is permitted, as are spirits—like scotch, rye, vodka and gin—with ice or no-calorie mixers.

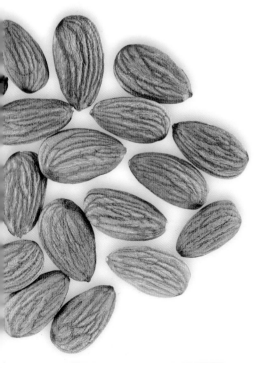

THE PROS

• Some research has found that following a low-carb diet helped people lose weight faster (and maintain that weight loss) than eating a low-fat diet. But the number of daily carbs—and types—isn't consistent and some people have had more success than others.

• "Staying away from high-sugar foods and beverages and increasing water intake is a good way to help regulate blood sugar levels," says Jeanette Kimszal, R.D.N.

THE CONS

• Carbs aren't evil. They're in vegetables, fruits, legumes, whole-grain foods, dairy products and many of the foods you eat for energy.

• Like with many other low-carb plans, you may miss out on fiber, says Mascha Davis, R.D.N., "which is actually one of the best things you can eat." Whole grains and fiber can help reduce your risk of cardiovascular diseases, as well as help you control your weight.

• Don't fall into the habit of eating processed bars, shakes and frozen meals. Many contain sugar alcohols, which can have a laxative effect on your GI tract.

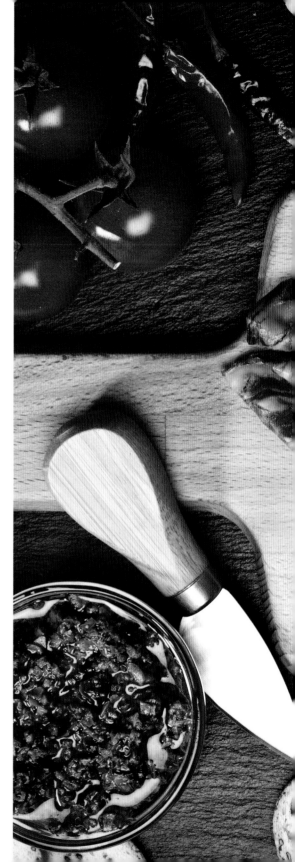

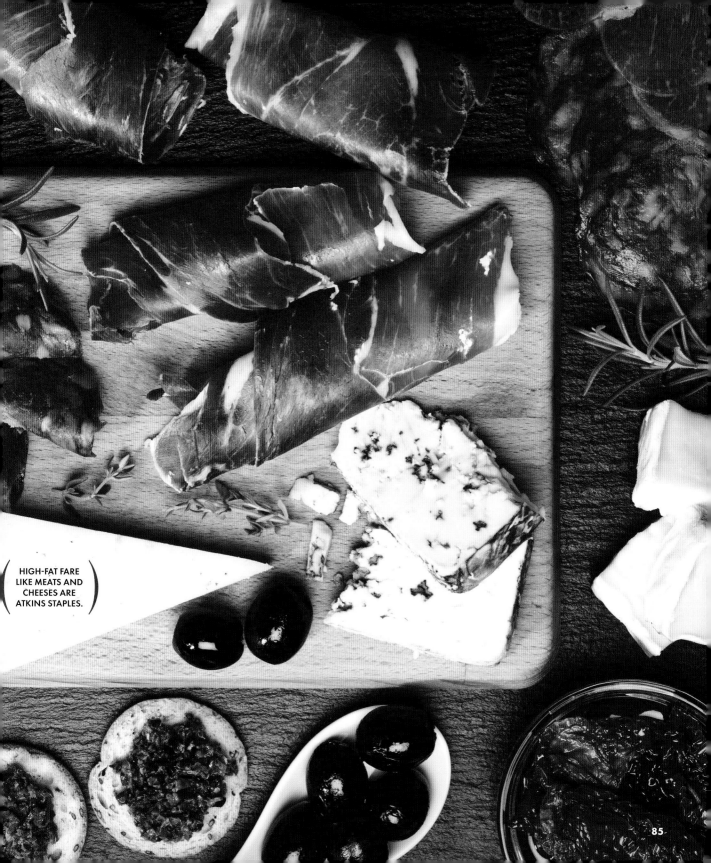

HIGH-FAT FARE LIKE MEATS AND CHEESES ARE ATKINS STAPLES.

Bone Broth Diet

If you really love soups and broths, you might be able to make it through this three-week intermittent-fasting plan.

What Is It?

This 21-day eating plan is a combination of the Paleo way of eating and intermittent fasting. Plus, you'll consume bone broth every day of the diet, so get ready to drink up!

Even though it may seem like a recent trend, the woman who is credited with kick-starting this diet—Kellyann Petrucci, M.S., N.D., author of *Dr. Kellyann's Bone Broth Diet: Lose Up to 15 Pounds, 4 Inches—and Your Wrinkles!—in Just 21 Days!*—says that she's been prescribing this plan to patients for years.

How It Works

Although there are different versions of bone broth diets, we'll focus on Petrucci's plan. You'll eat three Paleo Diet–friendly meals, five days a week, and stop all food consumption by 7 p.m. On two (nonconsecutive) days you'll consume only bone and vegetable broth about six times a day. You'll lose weight—and probably quickly—but that's likely due to calorie restriction, experts believe. That being said, there is quite a bit of research that associates a number of health benefits with intermittent fasting, such as blood sugar regulation.

What You'll Eat

You'll consume a variety of lean proteins, healthy fats and nonstarchy vegetables for three meals, supplemented with bone broth. Unlike regular consommé, bone broth is made from animal bones (usually chicken or beef) that have been boiled for six to 12 hours to make a homemade, collagen-packed soup. The broth itself delivers an excellent amount of satiating protein, vitamins and minerals, says Amy Gorin, M.S., R.D.N., and owner of Amy Gorin Nutrition in the New York City area. Even better, it's been credited with helping to provide a number of health benefits, from healing one's gut to weight loss to improving your immune system, as well as helping you look younger.

Foods to Avoid

Stay away from sugar, dairy, grains, gluten, processed foods and alcohol because the diet says these foods cause inflammation.

THE PROS

- "Bone broth can be a healthy part of a balanced diet," says Amy Gorin, M.S., R.D.N. It provides lots of nutrients with few calories.

- Eliminating processed foods can reduce inflammation and help you drop excess pounds.

- If you want to lose weight quickly, this is the diet for you. While the first few pounds are probably water weight, that's OK if you just want to fit into your favorite jeans by Saturday.

THE CONS

- "Neither Paleo nor intermittent fasting diets are what I recommend to clients," says Gorin. "I would suggest following an eating plan that doesn't cut out nutritious foods like legumes, grains, gluten and dairy."

- This plan will be particularly challenging to follow on fasting days, and you may get so hungry that you overeat.

- "I don't like that the diet punishes you for slipping—if you eat any of the restricted foods, you have to start all over," says Gorin.

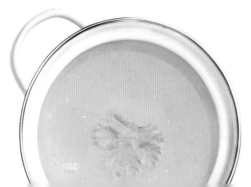

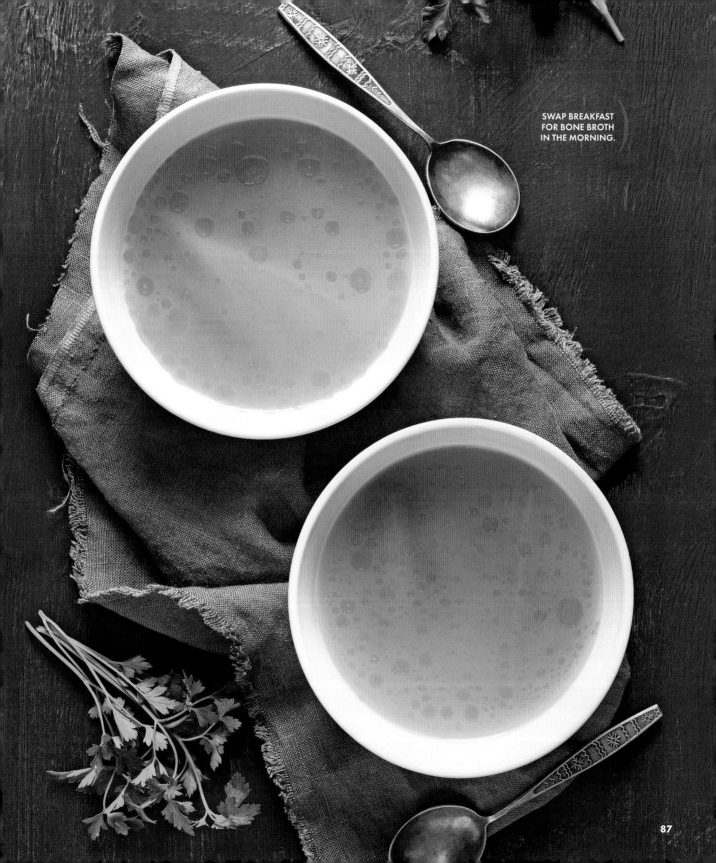

SWAP BREAKFAST
FOR BONE BROTH
IN THE MORNING.

87

Carb Cycling Diet

On the laundry list of carb-centric diets, this one takes the cake for the most lenient of dieters.

What Is It?

This trending carb-cutting diet switches things up and takes a different approach to manipulating carb intake. Carb cycling involves alternating your carbohydrate intake on a daily or weekly basis. "It's a strategy that involves eating higher amounts of carbohydrates on certain days of the week and doing the opposite—restricting carbs to low levels—on the other days," explains Josh Axe, D.N.M., C.N.S., D.C., founder of Ancient Nutrition and draxe.com. For example, a 160-pound, sedentary woman who is eating about 1,800 calories per day might eat 200 grams of carbs on one day and then drop down to 80 grams when carb cycling.

How It Works

The main goal of carb cycling is to match your body's need for energy, or glucose, with your diet. So, when your glucose demands are less—i.e., during periods of less activity—you limit or cut out your carb intake to, say, 25 percent of total caloric intake. "This can be done during the day by just consuming some carbs early or right before a workout. Or it can be done on a weekly basis, if your activity levels are greater on the weekend, for example," explains Roger Adams, Ph.D., C.P.T., owner of eatrightfitness.com. "When you carb cycle, [most] calories are made up of lean protein and healthy fats."

What You'll Eat

Axe recommends that you choose nutrient-dense carbs that provide vitamins, minerals and fiber whenever possible. In other words, carb cycling shouldn't be viewed as an excuse to binge-eat sweets and junk food! "Foods that

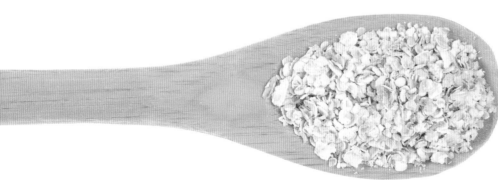

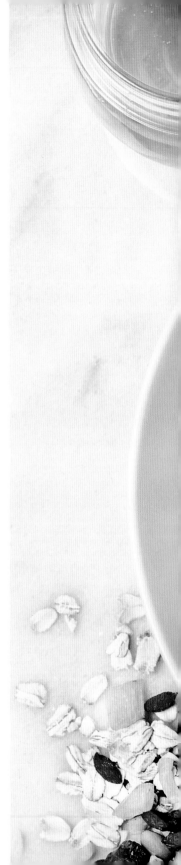

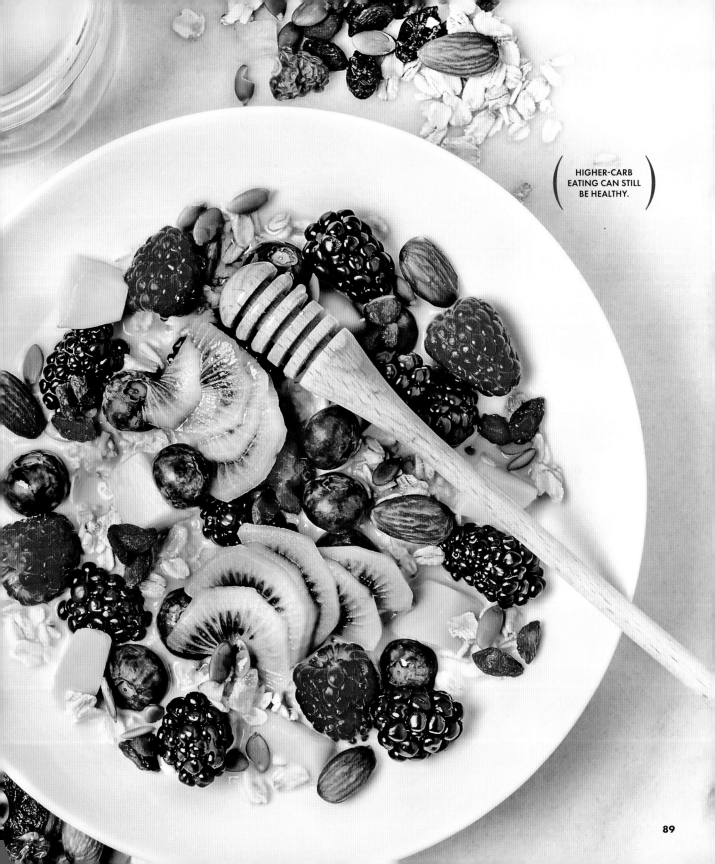

HIGHER-CARB
EATING CAN STILL
BE HEALTHY.

should provide the bulk of your carbohydrates include a variety of fruits, whole grains, dairy, beans/legumes and all types of vegetables," he says. "On lower-carb days, nonstarchy veggies, grass-fed meats, eggs, fish and healthy fats/oils should be the base of your meals."

Foods to Avoid

Foods that should be eaten in limited amounts include breads and other foods made with processed grains, like pasta, sweetened snacks and pizza.

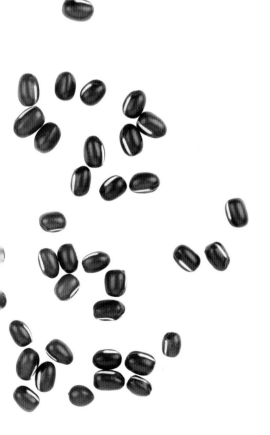

THE PROS

• "With a focus on whole foods, high fiber or lower-sugar fruits, and healthy fats, this can be a healthy diet," says Roger Adams, Ph.D., C.P.T. It keeps your metabolism running at a healthy pace.

• "Carb cycling is good for weight loss, a high metabolism, helping with athletic performance and muscle gains and recovery," says Josh Axe, D.N.M., C.N.S., D.C.

THE CONS

• Go into it with the expectation that you may experience temporary side effects like cravings, low energy, indigestion or thirst. "Side effects from low-carb eating are most likely to occur if it's a very different way of eating from what you're accustomed to," says Axe.

• In order to be successful, you need to plan out your week in advance, says Axe. Look at where social events fall, and plan for those to be higher-carb days. While carb cycling allows for flexibility, it does involve being less spontaneous and intuitive with food than you're used to. It may still feel restrictive at times.

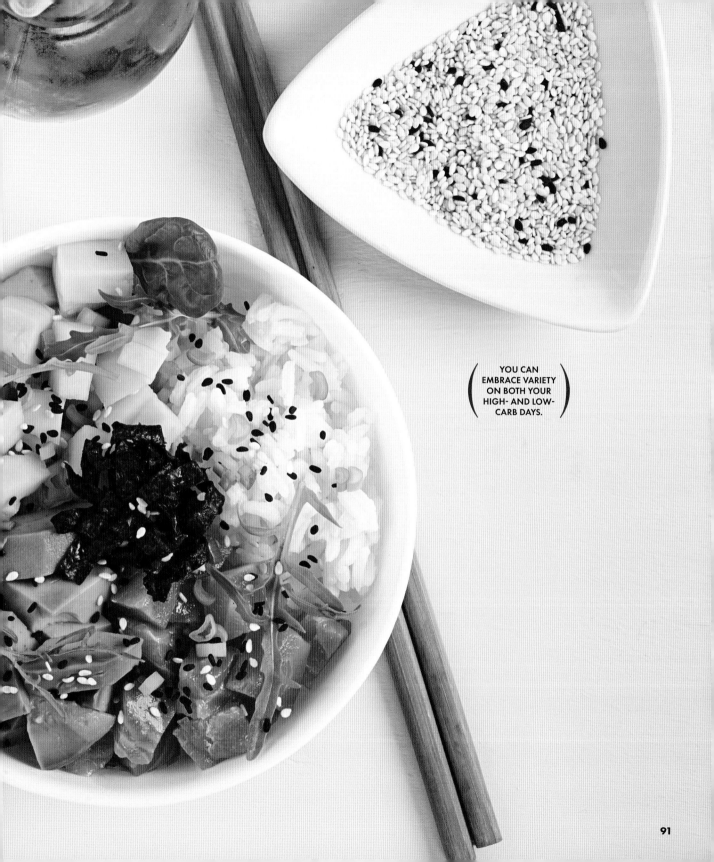

YOU CAN
EMBRACE VARIETY
ON BOTH YOUR
HIGH- AND LOW-
CARB DAYS.

The DASH Diet

When you're ready to make small changes that add up to better overall health as well as weight loss, this diet can help.

What Is It?

This eating and exercise plan was created by the National Heart, Lung, and Blood Institute and labeled the Dietary Approaches to Stop Hypertension (DASH).

While the diet started out as a way to lower blood pressure, it also lowers the risk of heart disease, cancer and diabetes, and can be used to lose weight, says Megan Casper, M.S., R.D.N., and owner of Nourished Bite. Eating a diet rich in fruits, vegetables and whole grains, and low in added sugar, sodium and processed meats, slows aging and helps you lose weight. *U.S. News & World Report* ranked The DASH Diet the No. 1 diet for eight years. "I regularly recommend this eating style to my clients, many of whom do not have high blood pressure," says Casper.

How It Works

Yes, it's designed to have specific heart-healthy outcomes—but it is relatively easy to follow, once you have a grasp of which foods are healthiest and which ones to stay away from. The food recommendations were originally derived to help people with high blood pressure, but they can help everyone lead a healthy lifestyle and lose weight slowly, says Casper. Your daily calorie range—anywhere from 1,600 to 3,000—depends on your gender, age and activity level. Find detailed guidelines on the National Heart, Lung, and Blood Institute's website: nhlbi.nih.gov/health-topics/dash-eating-plan.

What You'll Eat

DASH focuses on consuming plenty of whole grains, legumes, vegetables, fruit, low-fat animal products (lean meats, poultry, fish) and nonfat or low-fat dairy products. Eating a diet rich in plant-based foods is shown to help lower your risk for obesity, cancers, heart disease and more. This diet is about eating in a way that can be made into a lasting lifestyle, says Casper. "To get started, try adding one more serving of vegetables at lunch or dinner, use half the amount of butter you usually do, add a piece of fruit as a snack, try new spices and drink an extra glass of water."

Foods to Avoid

This diet is lower in salt, fat, added sugars, refined carbs and red meat than the typical American diet. No food is off-limits, but try to avoid high-fat foods like fatty meats and full-fat dairy, sweets and high-salt foods. Keep sodium to less than 2,300 mg daily.

THE PROS

- Reducing sodium decreases your risk of heart disease, high blood pressure and stroke. It also helps you de-bloat, so your clothes fit better and your stomach looks flatter.

- The DASH Diet does not require drastic changes. You can begin with small shifts, such as adding a serving of veggies to each meal or going for a 15-minute walk.

- The DASH Diet is lower in fat than the typical Western diet, so it's both heart-healthy and weight-friendly.

THE CONS

- The National Institutes of Health recommends taking it slow and adding small changes to ease into this diet, says Megan Casper, M.S., R.D.N. While that's not a bad thing, if you're looking for a diet with wham-bam weight-loss results in a week, this probably isn't it.

- DASH limits fat to less than 30 percent of total calories and encourages fat-free and low-fat fare, which can be less satisfying than products with more dietary fat.

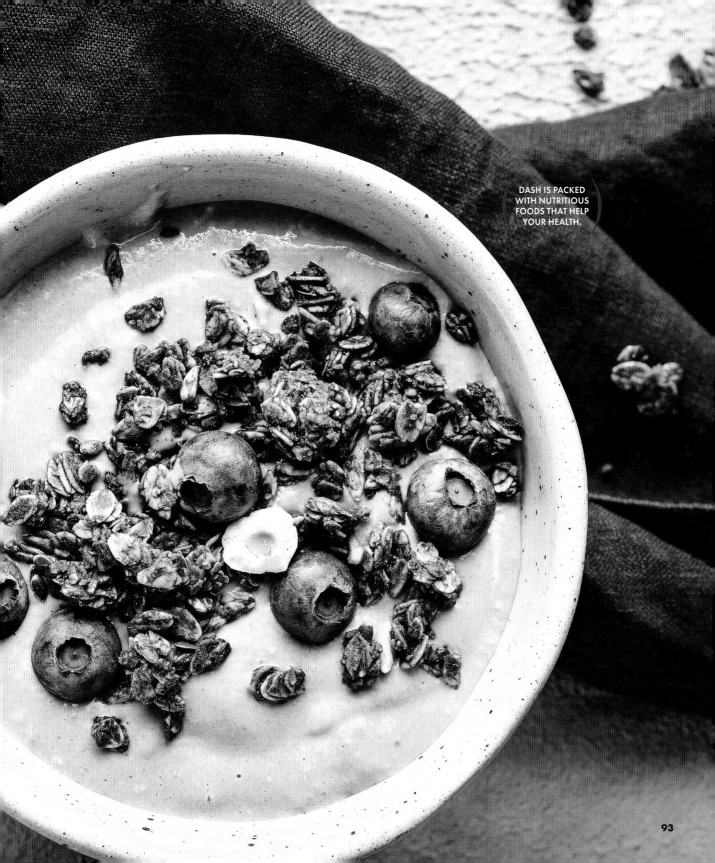

DASH IS PACKED
WITH NUTRITIOUS
FOODS THAT HELP
YOUR HEALTH.

Dr. Gundry's Diet Evolution

This three-phase plan is designed to restrict your diet to "trick" your genes so you can lose weight and get healthier.

What Is It?

Former heart surgeon Steven Gundry, M.D., was obese and insulin-resistant, even though he worked out daily and ate "healthy." He studied the underlying causes of heart disease, diabetes and obesity and then created this diet plan. His 2008 book of the same name focuses on altering your diet to outsmart your genes and lose weight.

How It Works

Gundry claims that foods usually thought to be "good" for you are actually "bad" because they aren't beneficial to your overall health. Once your genes get what they want, they activate other "killer genes" that exist to get rid of individuals who have outlived their usefulness, according to Gundry's philosophy. In the diet's Teardown phase, you'll significantly change your eating habits to kick-start weight loss for six weeks. Then the six-week Restoration phase follows, with a hunter-gatherer lifestyle plan that "tricks" your genes into stopping the "killer" phase. The last phase, Longevity, can help add years to your life, Gundry claims.

What You'll Eat

The portion sizes of the "friendly" foods change with each phase. You'll need to follow the book to get it right. You can eat most meat, poultry, fish, dairy, nuts and seeds. Eat as many leafy greens as you want, as well as artichokes, beans, broccoli and mushrooms. You can eat certain fruits after the first phase, including apples, cherries, nectarines and strawberries, in limited quantities.

Foods to Avoid

On this plan, you must always avoid "white" and "beige" foods. You also avoid lectins (a plant protein found in many foods such as eggplant, tomatoes, lentils, beans and peanuts). Gundry's belief in the importance of avoiding lectins later led him to create The Plant Paradox Diet (page 126).

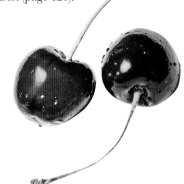

THE PROS

- Reducing your consumption of foods made with refined flour is a positive, says Michelle Dudash, R.D.N., author of *Clean Eating for Busy Families*. And the whole-grain versions are fine to eat after the first two weeks.

- Cutting back on animal products and cheese may be beneficial, says Dudash. Replacing animal foods with plants boosts fiber in your diet.

THE CONS

- While there is evidence that eliminating lectins from your diet can help certain diseases, it may not be advisable for everyone to ban entire food groups because they contain lectins, according to the Mayo Clinic.

- "A deprivation diet [like this] will help people lose weight in the short-term," says Dudash. "But this strict diet would be difficult to stick to, so you [might regain the weight]."

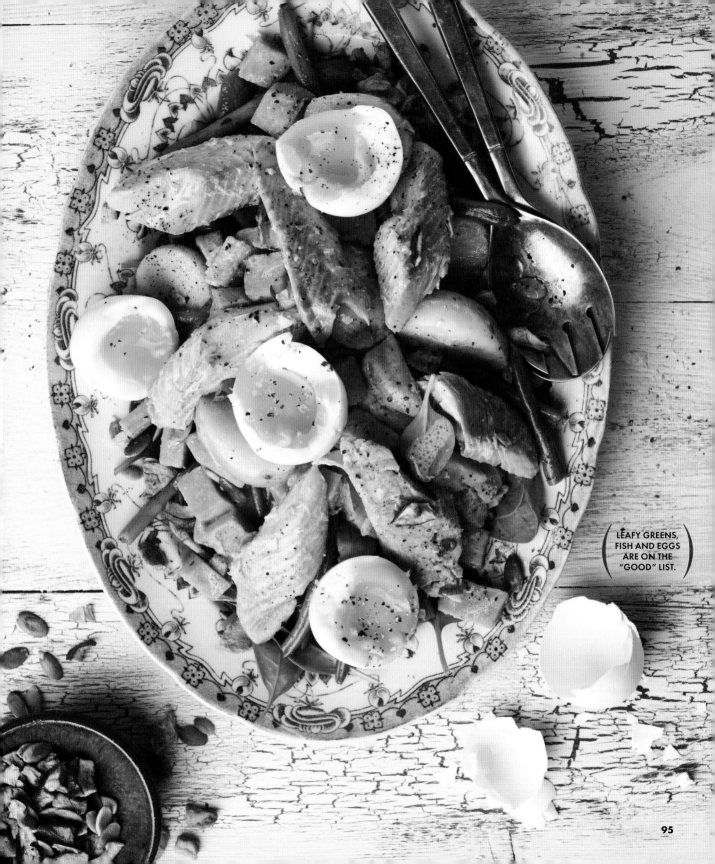

LEAFY GREENS, FISH AND EGGS ARE ON THE "GOOD" LIST.

The Dubrow Diet

The reality TV stars' interval plan is a lot like intermittent fasting—but with more food rules.

What Is It?

The Dubrow Diet is an interval-eating (intermittent-fasting) plan created by two reality TV stars: plastic surgeon Terry Dubrow, M.D., of *Botched*, and his wife, Heather Dubrow, formerly on *The Real Housewives of Orange County*. They say this way of eating trains the body to burn fat and lose weight.

During intermittent fasting, your body is forced to tap into stored fat for energy. You're improving the body's insulin response, as well as "resetting" the satiety center in the brain, the section that controls hunger levels. This is an area where there's a lot of research about the health benefits, says Carolyn Williams, Ph.D., R.D.

How It Works

Time-restricted eating allows for normal intake of food within a specific time frame, followed by a fasting interval, says Rachel Swanson, R.D.N. There are three phases to this diet: Red-Carpet Ready (16-hour fast, eight-hour refuel) followed by two to five days of specific food rules. The second phase, Summer Is Coming, gives options of three interval-eating schedules to follow: 12/12 fast/refuel; 14/10 fast/refuel; or 16/8 fast/refuel. Your own goals and how fast you want to lose weight will determine what intervals to follow; shorter feeding intervals will result in faster weight loss.

What You'll Eat

During refuel hours, you'll eat a lower-carb, clean-eating meal plan. When Williams followed The Dubrow Diet, she documented her macros. A Phase 1 day had 912 calories, 94 grams protein and 63 grams carbs. On a Phase 2 day, Williams ate 1,100 calories, with 95 grams of protein and 83 grams of carbs. The diet mostly focuses on lean proteins and green vegetables as well as specific fruits, complex carbs and healthy fats.

Foods to Avoid

You'll be limited to certain dairy choices (like mozzarella, ricotta, 2 percent milk and 2 percent Greek yogurt) and need to limit starchy carbs. Sugars are discouraged, as are processed foods. That being said, there are cheat snacks, meals and days that you can add in weekly to enjoy your favorite foods.

THE PROS

- If you don't want to count calories and carbs or eliminate entire food groups, you might like eating this way once you get a handle on the list of foods recommended during the "Summer Is Coming" phase.

- There's an intuitive-eating component to this plan.

- Alcohol is allowed. (Heather Dubrow is a big fan of Champagne!)

- You'll probably lose weight, and quickly, if you follow the 16/8 plan, while improving hunger levels.

- Intermittent fasting can help with energy levels.

THE CONS

- "This diet was pretty restrictive during the metabolism reset phase and even the Summer Is Coming phase. The daily calories were below 1,200," says Carolyn Williams, Ph.D., R.D.

- Some parts of the book emphasize somewhat superficial benefits, like looking good in a bikini, which can create an unhealthy body image.

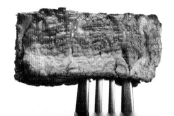

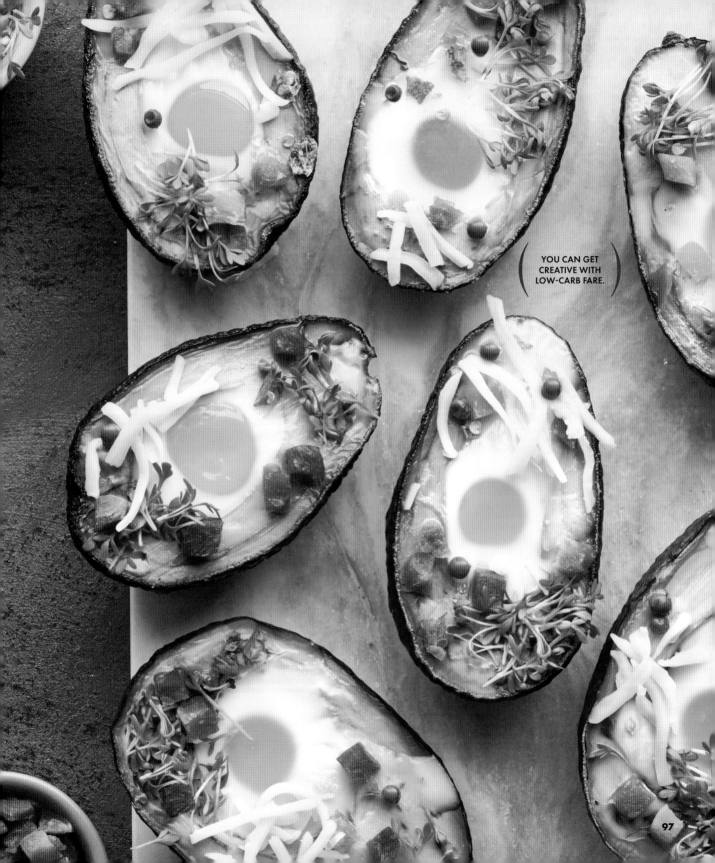

YOU CAN GET CREATIVE WITH LOW-CARB FARE.

97

The F-Factor Diet

This high-fiber diet is based on the premise that feeling fuller can ultimately help you eat less and lose more weight.

What Is It?

This diet and the book, *The F-Factor Diet: Discover the Secret to Permanent Weight Loss*, were created by registered dietitian Tanya Zuckerbrot, with its main component of fiber (the F) being the weight-loss secret. Fiber is a type of carbohydrate, but it's indigestible—which helps make you feel full without added calories, says Courtney Anaya, M.S., L.D.N., creator of The Food Fix. The diet plan evolved from Zuckerbrot's work with patients to improve cholesterol or control diabetes. She noticed they tended to lose weight without hunger by eating a diet rich in fiber. Eating the "right" carbs can help rev your metabolism, the diet claims. The F-Factor Diet encourages high-fiber foods and dining out and allows alcohol consumption.

How It Works

One of the main goals of the diet is to educate individuals on the right foods they should be eating, says Anaya. This is a plan centered on adding the right (fiber-rich) foods to your diet rather than eliminating certain choices. Like many plans outlined in this book, this diet is broken down into three phases. During Step 1, you'll have fewer than 35 grams of net carbs (total grams of carbs minus grams of fiber) daily for two weeks. You'll stay under 75 grams net carbs for Step 2, until you reach your goal. Finally, in the maintenance phase, Step 3, you'll aim for around 125 grams net carbs. Choosing foods that are high in fiber, so your net carbs are lower, is what this diet is all about.

What You'll Eat

Fiber-based foods that you can eat during the first two weeks include some fruits and nonstarchy vegetables and homemade baked goods with a high-fiber protein powder. Going into the second stage of the diet, your net carbs will increase, with three more servings of carbs daily. Fruit, whole-grain pasta and whole-wheat bread can be explored during Step 2. The goal is to see continued weight loss during this phase.

Foods to Avoid

Certain foods (starchy vegetables, starches, fruits) are skipped during Step 1 to accelerate weight loss, but are added back in Step 2.

THE PROS

- This diet puts the focus back on fiber and the health benefits that come with it, not just weight loss, says Courtney Anaya, M.S., L.D.N. "Increased fiber intake has been linked to stabilizing blood sugar levels, reducing the risk of developing some cancers and enhancing energy levels."

- You can dine out and drink alcohol on this plan.

THE CONS

- You'll still need to calculate and track carbs during this diet's weight-loss phases, so if you're someone who hates tracking, this plan might not be best for you.

- Going into the second stage, where the net carb and fiber intake is increased, gassiness and bloating may occur, advises Anaya. "This can happen because it's not a gradual increase. Listen to your body and adjust the carb intake, if needed, in this phase."

- Eating high-fiber, processed foods that are low-carb and have sugar alcohols can wreak havoc on your digestive system.

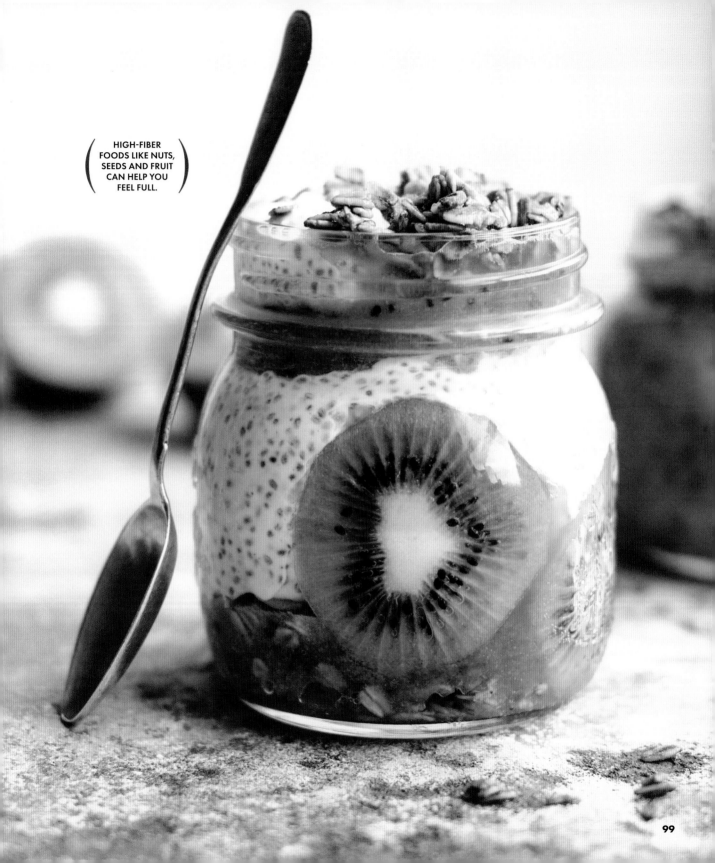

HIGH-FIBER FOODS LIKE NUTS, SEEDS AND FRUIT CAN HELP YOU FEEL FULL.

The Flexitarian Diet

*This semivegetarian eating approach
may be a great fit for people who don't
want to commit to a strict or restrictive diet.*

What Is It?

The flexitarian diet comes from a combo of the words "flexible" and "vegetarian." Also called semivegetarianism, it means eating primarily vegetarian, with the occasional inclusion of meat and other animal products.

The word flexitarian has been around since about 1998, but it became more popular once Dawn Jackson Blatner, L.D.N., wrote *The Flexitarian Diet* in 2008. For the past five years, it has consistently ranked near the top of the *U.S. News & World Report*'s "Best Diets Overall" rankings as one of the best overall diets and one of the easiest to follow.

How It Works

You'll eat a more plant-based diet by ramping up your intake of fruits, vegetables, legumes and whole grains—without eliminating any foods from your diet. "A flexitarian diet is, by definition, very flexible," says Julieanna Hever, M.S., R.D., C.P.T., author of *Plant-Based Nutrition*. Beginners should aim for seven meatless meals per week; advanced followers should try for eight to 14.

What You'll Eat

You'll include more plant-based proteins (such as lentils and beans), whole grains, potatoes, fruit, vegetables, cow and plant milks, eggs and healthy fats (such as olive oil, avocados and fish like salmon). In her book, Blatner describes a typical day's meal plan: avocado toast, spinach and an egg for breakfast; a kale bowl with chicken or chickpeas, tomatoes, roasted sweet potato and dressing for lunch; tacos with white fish or lentils, corn tortillas, slaw, guacamole and salsa for dinner.

Foods to Avoid

You don't need to ditch meat and dairy completely, but as a flexitarian, you'll cut back on poultry, red meat and pork, as well as animal fats, like butter and cheese. Some flexitarians limit meat to one or two days a week; others eat vegan for most of the day, then have meat or poultry for dinner—it's up to you. You'll also eliminate or cut back on processed foods, sweets and foods with added sugar.

THE PROS

- Research has found that flexitarian diets may help reduce body weight, improve metabolic health and blood pressure, and reduce the risk of Type 2 diabetes. It may even play a role in treating inflammatory bowel diseases.

- The diet's flexibility could make it a great choice for helping to develop healthy eating habits you can maintain for life, especially if you don't want to cut out any foods.

THE CONS

- Eliminating animal products can put you at risk for some nutrient deficiencies. "The most common are iron, zinc, calcium, vitamin D, B12 and omega-3 fats," says Dawn Jackson Blatner, L.D.N. (Note: You can get these in plant foods, through a combo of whole grains, legumes, vegetables, nuts and seeds, except for vitamin B12, which you can get through fortified foods or a supplement.)

- The benefits aren't as noticeable as a vegan diet, says Neal Barnard, M.D. "You may not lose weight as fast, which can make you discouraged."

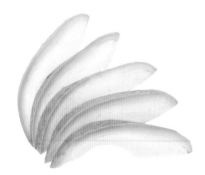

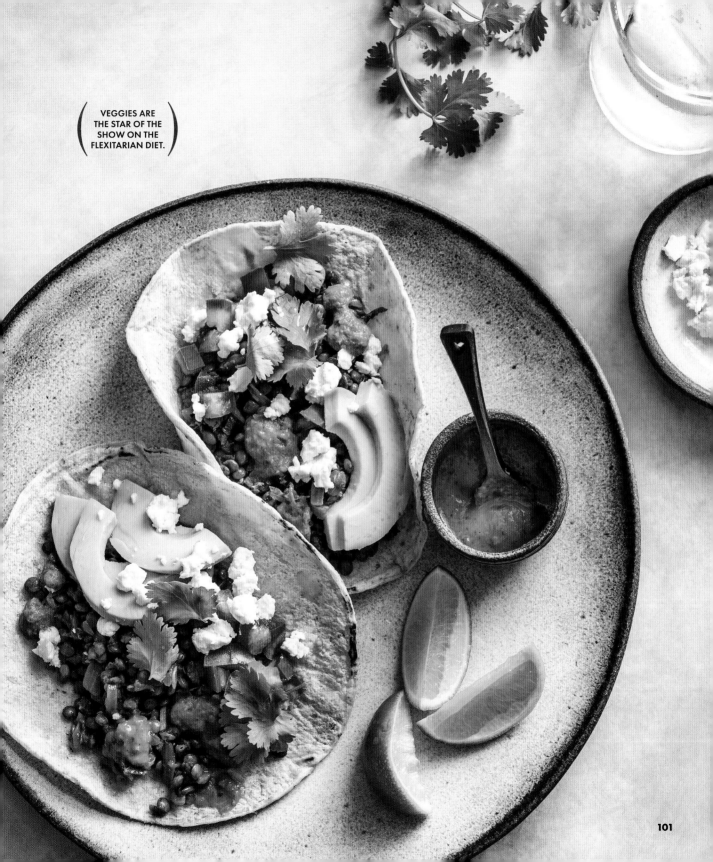

VEGGIES ARE
THE STAR OF THE
SHOW ON THE
FLEXITARIAN DIET.

101

Intermittent Fasting Diet

Also known as the 5:2 Diet or The Fast Diet, this plan involves two low-calorie days a week, mixed in with five "normal" days of eating.

What Is It?

The Fast Diet is a low-calorie intermittent-fasting weight-loss plan co-created by Michael Mosley, a medical journalist who trained as a doctor at the Royal Free Hospital in London, and *Evening Standard* journalist Mimi Spencer. It's often referred to as the 5:2 Diet because you eat as you normally would five days a week, and restrict your calories on two nonconsecutive days a week to just 25 percent of your daily needs. (That's roughly 600 calories a day for men and 500 calories a day for women.)

How It Works

Research suggests that modified-fasting regimens can result in weight loss and lead to metabolic improvements, even improving insulin sensitivity in those who are diagnosed with Type 2 diabetes, says Rachel Swanson, M.S., R.D., L.D.N., founder of RachelsRx. Although subsisting on just 500 or 600 calories sounds miserable, Mosley claims that his hunger pangs subsided quicker than he expected. He also felt that fasting sharpened his wits and helped him feel more focused.

FIBER-RICH FRUITS AND VEGETABLES ARE ON THE MENU ON LOW-CALORIE DIET DAYS.

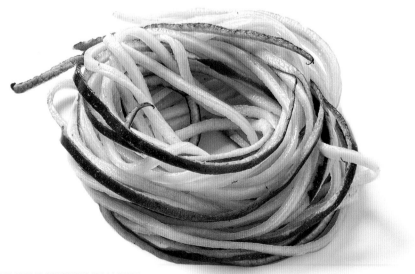

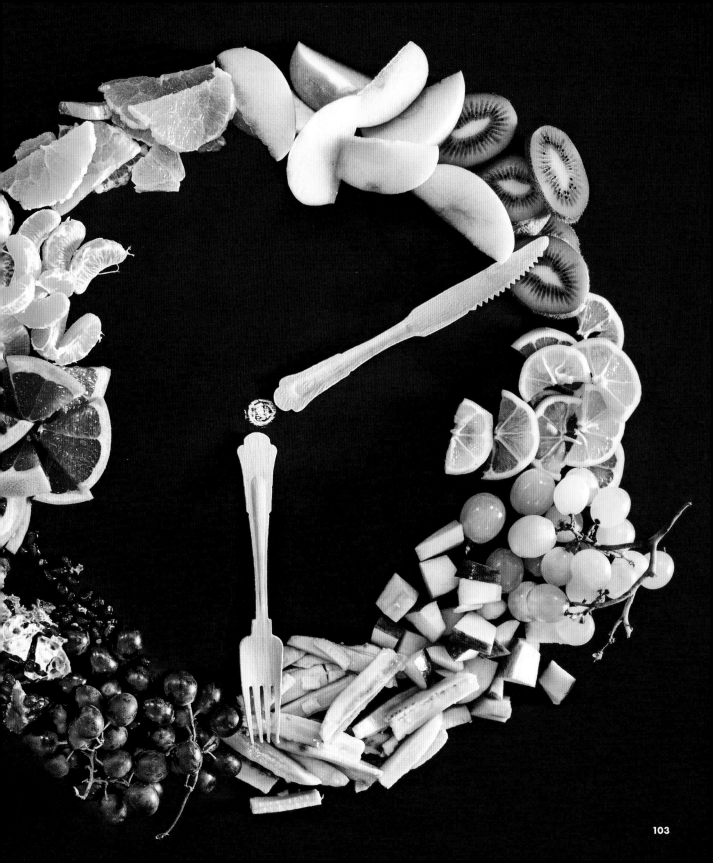

What You'll Eat

Eat what you want on normal eating days—just stick to the recommended calorie range. You'll have better health benefits if you focus on consuming wholesome foods rather than processed ones. On low-calorie days, you should consume high-protein fare like chicken, fish, tofu, nuts, eggs and legumes to help keep you feeling fuller for longer, as well as fiber-rich, low-calorie fruits and vegetables. You can consume your 500 or 600 calories all in one meal, or simply have several snacks throughout the day.

Foods to Avoid

No food is off-limits on this diet plan, but that is not an invitation to pig out. Adhere to the daily calorie rules for best results.

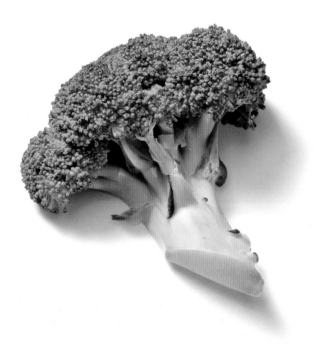

THE PROS

• You can choose which days work best for your calorie restriction.

• "Time-restricted eating is a great 'first step' for anyone who is not yet fully engaged or committed to change their dietary behavior," suggests Rachel Swanson, M.S., R.D., L.D.N.

• There are no costs involved in following The Fast Diet. You don't have to overhaul your pantry or refrigerator with new ingredients, and you may even save money on fasting days, since you'll be eating much less.

THE CONS

• The Fast Diet may not be practical for everyone, since it may lead to intense hunger on fasting days.

• If you have diabetes, consult your doctor before trying The Fast Diet—you may need to adjust your medications, since the drop in caloric intake could put you at risk for hypoglycemia.

• You'll need to stay organized and plan ahead for the week to decide which days are going to be your fasting days (those with fewer social plans) and when you're going to eat normally.

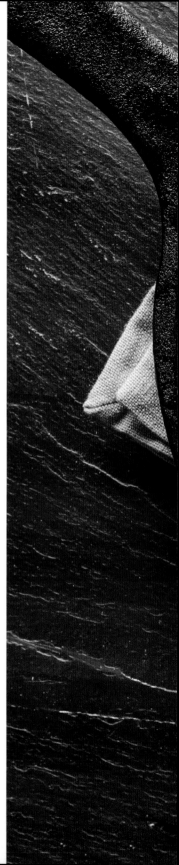

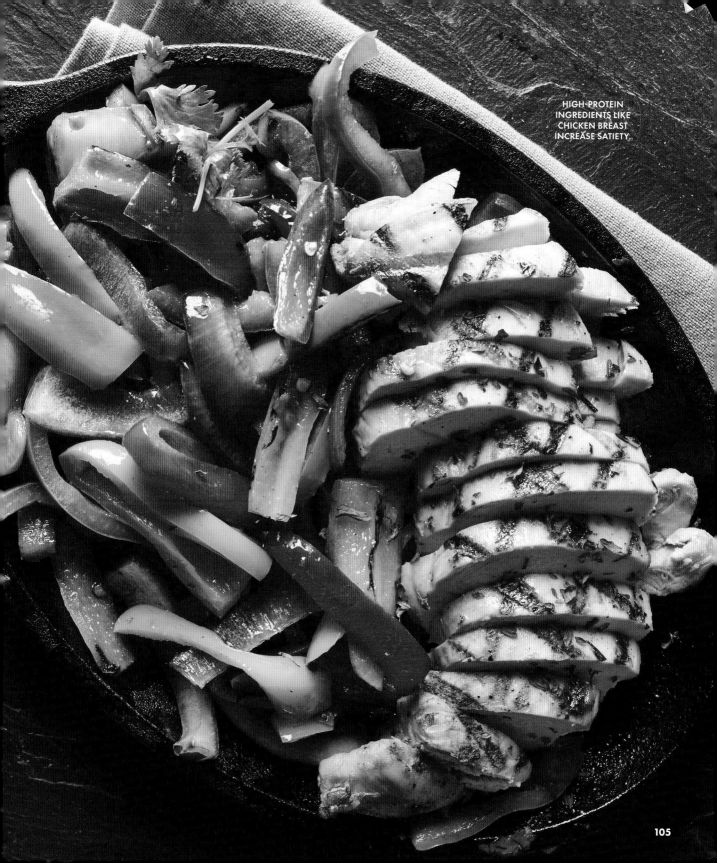

HIGH-PROTEIN
INGREDIENTS LIKE
CHICKEN BREAST
INCREASE SATIETY.

Intuitive Eating Diet

This way of eating teaches you how to tune in to your body's hunger and fullness signals so you can lose weight without giving up your favorite foods.

What Is It?

You won't have to follow a meal plan or count macros, and you can enjoy favorite foods on the intuitive eating diet. "There are no forbidden foods or calorie counting with the diet-free lifestyle approach of intuitive eating," says Eliza Kingsford, L.C.P., author of *Brain-Powered Weight Loss*. IE, as it's called, teaches you how to tune in to your body's signals of what true hunger and fullness really are.

How It Works

Dietitians Evelyn Tribole and Elyse Resch created IE in 1995, with the hope of breaking the cycle of chronic dieting. They developed 10 intuitive-eating principles:

1 Reject the diet mentality.
2 Honor your hunger.
3 Make peace with food.
4 Challenge the food police.
5 Feel your fullness.
6 Discover the satisfaction factor.
7 Cope with your emotions without using food.
8 Respect your body.
9 Exercise: Feel the difference.
10 Honor your health with nutrition.

"Although there is no set macronutrient/calorie requirement for IE, reliance is solely based on addressing one's hunger and fullness cues and distancing oneself from any 'faux' hunger or fullness that is intruded on by emotional/cognitive factors," says Monica Auslander Moreno, M.S., R.D.N. "You'll learn to know precisely when you are hungry and when you are full."

Most chronic dieters who engage in IE do see weight loss, because they were previously restricting and bingeing in a cycle that fosters weight gain. This isn't a quick weight-loss plan where you'll notice results in a week. It's about learning healthy practices to follow for a lifetime.

What You'll Eat

"You give yourself permission to eat whatever you want on this plan," says Kingsford. "This doesn't necessarily mean eating all junk food. The goal is to become mindful or intuitive about what your body needs, and the emphasis should be on whole foods, like vegetables and fruit."

Foods to Avoid

Although "all foods are allowed," Moreno discourages followers from eating foods that don't promote good health: "Soda, juice, candy and junk food should be avoided—but one food doesn't ruin a healthy way of eating."

THE PROS

• You'll get to a healthy weight; you'll have increased body trust and satisfaction and contentment, since no foods are forbidden.

• A trickle-down effect is often increased with exercise, says Monica Auslander Moreno, M.S., R.D.N.

THE CONS

• Many people find the thought of allowing themselves "forbidden" foods uncomfortable and daunting, says Moreno.

• It is easy to overeat, especially when you first start IE, before you are truly in tune with your body's hunger and fullness sensors.

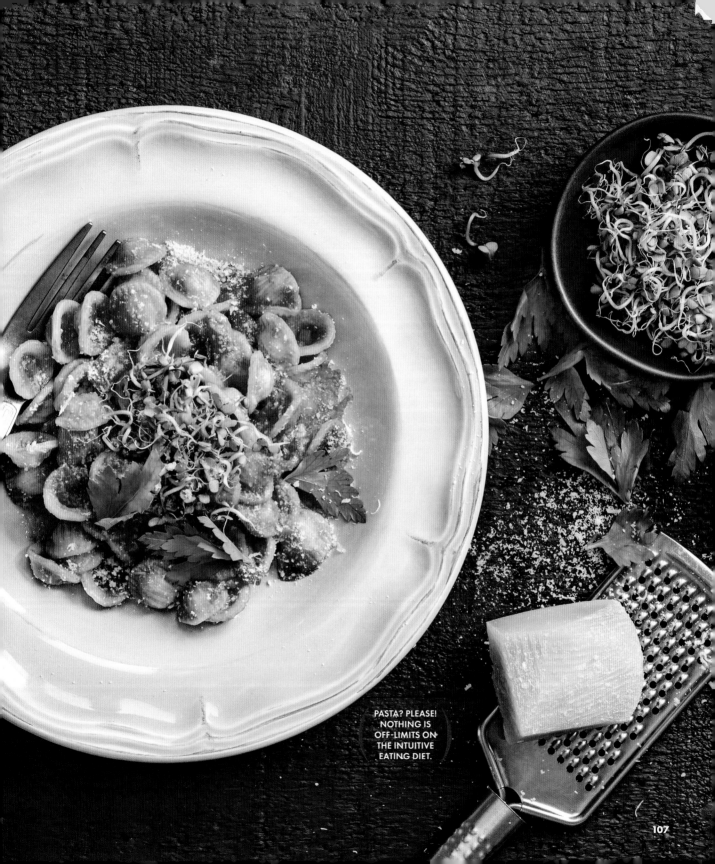

PASTA? PLEASE! NOTHING IS OFF-LIMITS ON THE INTUITIVE EATING DIET.

Juicing Diet

Ready to have all your meals through a straw? Find out whether this fruit- and vegetable-based diet is for you.

What Is It?

Chances are, someone in your inner circle has tried juicing at some point. Perhaps they did it to detox or jump-start weight loss after a vacation or holiday or to feel "lighter," as some followers claim.

"Juicing is a trend that has sustained itself beyond a momentary obsession," says Samina Kalloo, R.D., C.D.N. "Most [juicers] are trying to lose weight and get more nutrients."

How It Works

Following a juice diet means consuming a combination of mainly fruits and vegetables in liquid form.

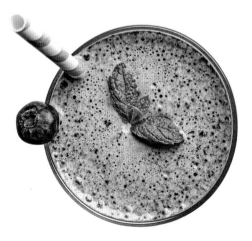

"Most juicing diets call for all meals and snacks to be replaced by juice and usually last from a few days to a few weeks," explains Kalloo. Since juice cleanses are often very low in calories, you'll likely experience a fast, initial weight loss. Most of that will be water weight, however—and it's also a result you would achieve on any similarly calorie-restrictive diet, she adds.

Advocates also believe it can help to detoxify and cleanse the body; however, there isn't enough published research to support these and other supposed health benefits, says Kalloo.

What You'll Eat

Ahem—we mean what you'll be drinking. Most cleanses involve drinking a few bottles of a fruit-and-vegetable juice blend, with a daily total that's usually around 1,200 to 1,300 calories. Some plans are three-day "cleanses" and others last weeks. While you can buy juices ready-made, you can also prepare them at home.

Foods to Avoid

A lot. Most juicing diets involve abstaining from all foods except for juice (from fruits and vegetables), water and herbal tea, says Kalloo.

THE PROS

- You'll lose weight quickly.

- A high intake of fruits and vegetables is linked to better weight management and a reduced risk of chronic diseases.

- One small study found subjects on a three-day juice cleanse experienced weight loss initially and during a two-week follow-up. They also had improvements to the intestinal microbiota associated with weight loss.

THE CONS

- Juice doesn't contain the fiber that whole fruits and vegetables do, which is what fills you up. You may end up bingeing.

- Since you're typically not consuming enough calories, your metabolism will likely slow down and you may have headaches and low energy.

- Juicing can be expensive and/or time-consuming.

- "All food groups contain micro- and macronutrients essential to health, so cutting out entire food groups can come with health concerns," says Samina Kalloo, R.D. The lack of protein can make it difficult to maintain muscle.

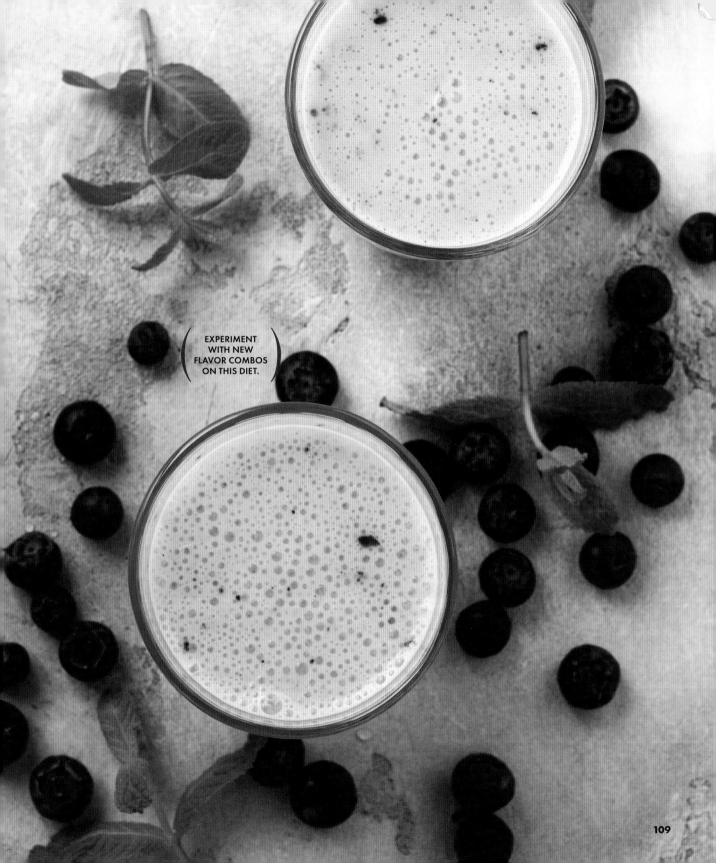

EXPERIMENT WITH NEW FLAVOR COMBOS ON THIS DIET.

The Keto Diet

The trendy ketogenic diet is all about eating a high-fat, low-carb diet to put your body into ketosis, a fat-burning mode.

What Is It?

You've probably heard the keto diet mentioned in the news, popularized by celebrities and Silicon Valley techies who claim that this way of eating helps them focus. "Keto" is short for ketosis, a metabolic process in the body. A keto diet is about 70 percent fat, 20 percent protein and 10 percent carbs. Because of this very low amount of carbs (less than 50 grams a day), your body mostly burns fat for fuel.

Although some keto-diet followers claim that eating this way can solve a range of health problems, from heart disease and diabetes to curing cancer and even autism, many health and nutrition experts don't necessarily agree, although more are getting on board with the plan.

Will you lose weight if you follow it? Yes. But it's an extreme diet that ranked last in the *U.S. News & World Report*'s "Best Diets Overall" roundup, which features input from a panel of health and nutrition experts.

How It Works

The ketogenic diet has been practiced since the 1920s and was originally designed to help epileptic patients reduce seizures, especially among children. In the ketosis state, the body's energy comes from ketone bodies in the blood. This metabolic state of burning fat instead of carbs for fuel is called ketosis. It takes about three to seven days—but sometimes a little longer—for your body to adjust to this process, and it often leads to a state known as the "keto flu." Symptoms can include tiredness, nausea, dizziness, difficulty concentrating, insomnia, an upset stomach, dehydration and funky-smelling breath (because your acetone levels increase when your body is in a state of ketosis).

"I don't like to say that something's dangerous, but I would just say that ketogenic is far [from healthy]," says Wesley Delbridge, R.D.N., a Phoenix-based spokesperson for the Academy of Nutrition and Dietetics. "I don't think a lot of people understand what's happening in their bodies."

But others say there are proven benefits. If you struggle to control yourself around carbs, this super-low-carb diet might help you rein in those carb cravings and keep blood sugar spikes in check. Keto is good for lowering and stabilizing blood sugar, since it naturally reduces sugar from the diet, says nutrition specialist Robert Silverman, D.C., M.S., C.N.S. "Good fats are

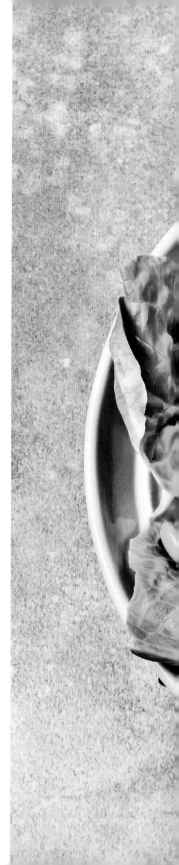

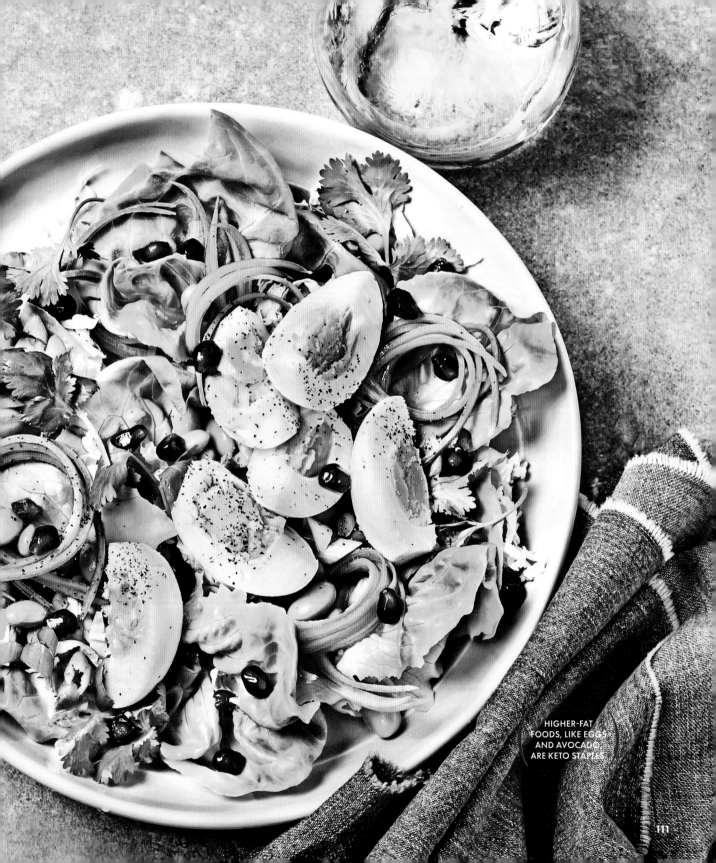

HIGHER-FAT
FOODS, LIKE EGGS
AND AVOCADO,
ARE KETO STAPLES

healthier for us; they make up our cell membrane and give us a sense of fullness," he says. "Most people think we get fullness from caloric intake, but we get it from efficient nutrients—you don't have to eat as many calories."

What You'll Eat

You'll mostly be eating high-fat, low-carb foods as well as nonstarchy vegetables and high-protein, low- or no-carb foods. On a typical keto diet shopping list you'll find eggs, olive oil, coconut oil, grass-fed butter, palm oil, macadamia nuts, seeds, grass-fed beef, spinach, tomatoes, chicken thighs, cheddar cheese, berries and cucumbers, as well as full-fat dairy products like yogurt, butter, heavy cream and sour cream. Protein should come from organic, grass-fed animal products whenever possible.

Foods to Avoid

There's a long list of foods to avoid that are thought to shut down your body's fat-burning ability. You won't be eating most fruits, starchy veggies, grains, legumes, beans and lighter dairy like low-fat yogurt on the keto diet. You'll also stay away from sugars and processed foods. Unhealthy fats include corn oil, soybean oil, canola oil, sesame oil, peanut oil, grapeseed oil and safflower oil.

Alcohol is predominantly a no-no on the keto diet, although spirits like vodka and whiskey are naturally low in carbs, so it's the mixers you need to be wary of. Of course, sweetened beverages are eliminated, too, including milk in your coffee (which is why some advocates recommend butter, ghee, heavy cream and/or coconut oil in their morning cup of Joe).

THE PROS

- Research has found that a keto diet can help you lose weight and reduce inflammation in the body. It can also lead to greater metabolic efficiency in consuming fats and may help protect against cognitive decline.

- "This way of eating usually has more people feeling fuller because all that fat really increases your satiety," says Wesley Delbridge, R.D.N. If you're feeling fuller, you'll eat less, which would translate to weight loss.

THE CONS

- The first few days on a keto diet might make you dizzy and lethargic. You may feel fuzzy because your brain runs on glucose, says Delbridge. "People report headaches, bad moods and fatigue." You may also develop breath that smells like nail polish remover.

- "People don't realize how few carbs they'll be eating," says Delbridge. "Some [keto] recommendations are for around 30 to 40 grams of carbs a day. That's about the equivalent of an apple or two slices of bread."

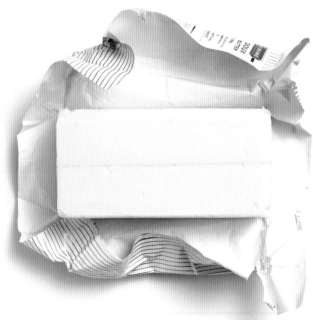

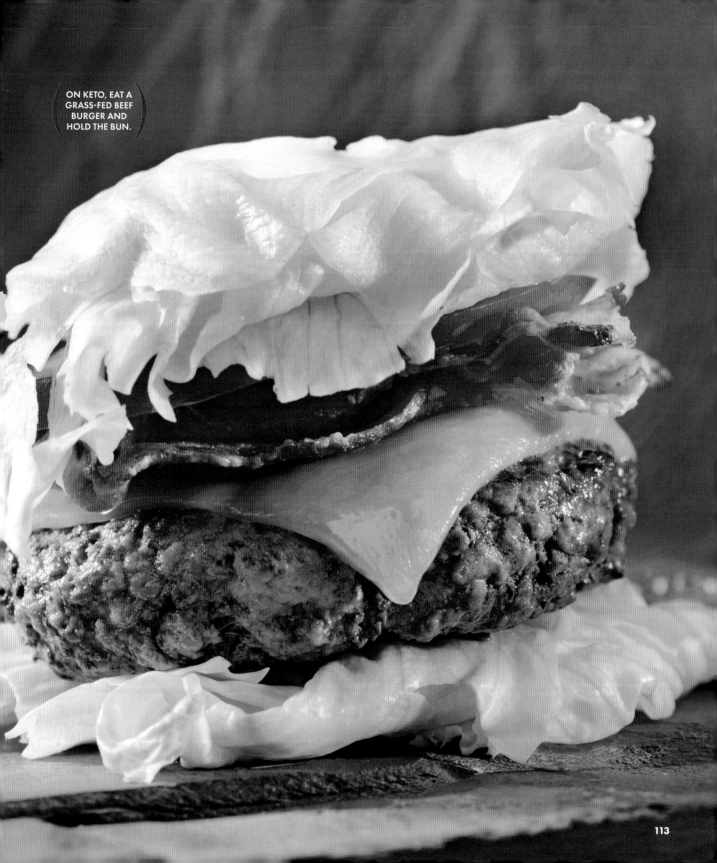

ON KETO, EAT A GRASS-FED BEEF BURGER AND HOLD THE BUN.

The Lose Your Belly Diet

TV talk-show host Dr. Travis Stork's diet focuses on gut health and overall well-being through whole foods that are nourishing, not restricting.

What Is It?

The human microbiome (all the tiny organisms that live in our bodies) has been an emerging area of research. *The Lose Your Belly Diet*—a 2017 book from Travis Stork, M.D., host of *The Doctors*—focuses on nourishing the gut microbiome to increase your chances of reaching a healthy weight and burning off belly fat.

How It Works

A healthy adult has many species of bacteria living in the large intestine, forming the microbiome. These bacteria help your body do everything from protecting your immunity to digesting food. "Researchers are now discovering that gut bacteria also seem to play a role in the complex process of weight loss and gain," Stork writes.

"Strengthening the gut microbiome helps diversify the bacteria in your body, helps with offenders and builds immunity," says Stacy K. Leung, R.D.N.

What You'll Eat

There's a heavy focus on high-fiber "prebiotics"—whole foods (onions, apples, jicama) that provide nutrients for gut bacteria to thrive. You'll eat unlimited fruits and vegetables; get protein from nuts, legumes, fish and dairy (limiting beef, pork and chicken as much as possible); and add even more fiber with whole grains. Healthy fats provide omega-3 fatty acids and help ward off hunger. You'll also eat at least one daily serving of a probiotic food, which contains living bacteria to help diversify and increase your gut bacteria. These include yogurt, kefir, kimchi, kombucha, miso and tempeh.

Foods to Avoid

No foods are banned outright, but a focus on whole foods means you'll skip refined foods, sugars and processed meats. Stork advocates buying organic foods and antibiotic-free animal products to avoid chemicals and antibiotics that harm the microbiome.

THE PROS

- You'll lose weight quickly.
- A high intake of fruits and vegetables is linked to better body-weight management, as well as a reduced risk of chronic diseases.

THE CONS

- "The gut microbiome is a very hot topic, but it needs more research," says Stacy K. Leung, R.D.N.
- While the book title focuses on belly fat, Stork doesn't promise you'll lose your belly with this plan. Instead, it's about raising your "chances of reaching and maintaining a healthy weight and burning off dangerous belly fat."
- Although you may save money by eating less meat, buying antibiotic- and hormone-free products as well as all organic foods could cause your grocery bill to increase.

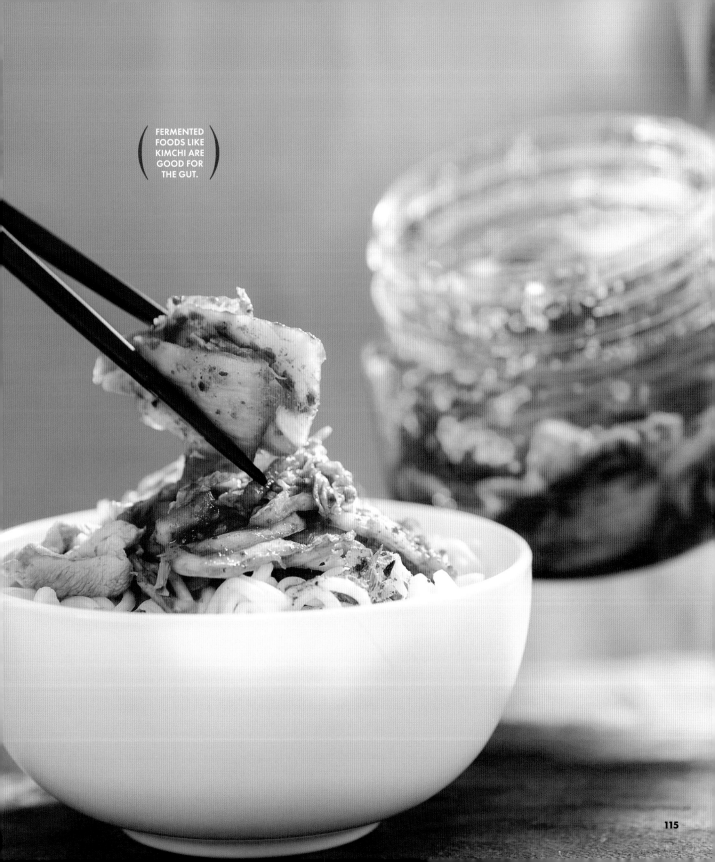

FERMENTED FOODS LIKE KIMCHI ARE GOOD FOR THE GUT.

Mediterranean Diet

This heart-healthy eating plan follows a lifestyle that you might enjoy no matter where you live.

What Is It?

Touted as one of the best eating plans by many nutrition and health experts, the Mediterranean diet predominantly relies on the traditional foods and cooking styles of countries bordering the Mediterranean Sea—think places like Italy, Spain, France, Greece, Israel and Lebanon.

"Those who embrace the Mediterranean lifestyle enjoy fresh, flavorful food made with quality ingredients," says Nancy Z. Farrell, R.D., an Academy of Nutrition and Dietetics spokeswoman based in Fredericksburg, Virginia. These cultural cuisines have historically been known to promote a healthy lifestyle, given their inclusion of large amounts of fresh produce (fruits and vegetables), whole grains, seafood and healthy fats.

How It Works

The Mediterranean diet focuses on consuming a variety of fresh foods in moderation, encouraging a wide array of produce, whole grains and lean proteins, which make up the majority of the menu. Basic tenets include enjoying fish and/ or seafood at least twice weekly and choosing nuts, poultry and low-fat dairy over red meat. Healthy fats, such as olive oil, avocado and nuts

(again!), in moderation, are also of paramount importance.

"This is really a centuries-long lifestyle approach to eating, and not a diet with a start and end date," Farrell says.

What You'll Eat

Try to eat about 10 servings of vegetables and fruits every day, says Farrell, who adds, "Make olive oil your go-to choice when fat is needed in cooking."

You'll also tend to enjoy eating more meatless meals. Farrell suggests incorporating beans, legumes, nuts and cheeses into meals, snacks and recipes. The same goes for selecting seafood—fish and shellfish—more often than processed and high-fat meats. Choosing these alternatives may also help to lower the level of LDL ("bad") cholesterol—the type that's more likely to build up deposits in your arteries, according to the Mayo Clinic website.

Experiment with a variety of whole grains, and "search out whole grains and millet and quinoa recipes," says Farrell.

One option that many followers enjoy: "Have a small glass of wine with dinner," suggests Farrell. (One study associated moderate consumption of ethanol, mostly from wine, with better survival.)

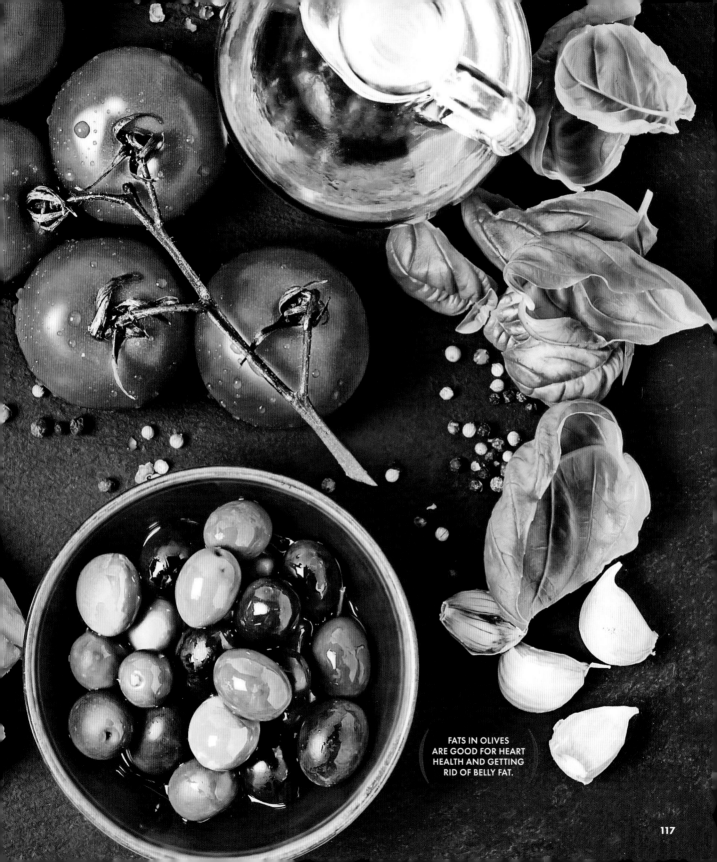

FATS IN OLIVES
ARE GOOD FOR HEART
HEALTH AND GETTING
RID OF BELLY FAT.

Foods to Avoid

Unlike with more restrictive diets, when following a Mediterranean "lifestyle" no foods are really considered to be off-limits. However, given the emphasis on whole foods and clean eating, it's best to avoid items that are refined, contain added sugars or are highly processed. That means limiting items such as soda and candy, as well as refined, non-whole grains (like in white bread or rice), processed meats and trans fats found in margarine.

In essence, the Mediterranean diet is all about eating fresh, whole foods and keeping an eye on your portion sizes while slowly savoring all of the flavors of your meals. "On a trip to Italy a few years ago, I enjoyed many a plate of al dente pasta at lunchtimes that enjoyably seemed to linger on," remembers Farrell.

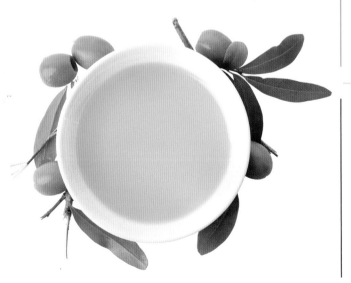

THE PROS

• Researchers love the diet's many health benefits. A number of studies have suggested that the Mediterranean lifestyle is effective in the reduction of chronic disease, namely heart disease.

• Research from a *New England Journal of Medicine* study indicates that following the guidelines of this diet may decrease the risk of heart disease and elevated blood pressure. According to research in the journal *Diabetes Care*, those at higher risk of developing Type 2 diabetes may also benefit from a Mediterranean eating pattern. Following this lifestyle may also lead to a reduction in metabolic syndrome.

THE CONS

• Requires frequent trips to the supermarket, significant meal prep and cooking.

• The diet does not offer specific guidelines or calorie counts. If you are looking for rules to follow, you may want to try another plan.

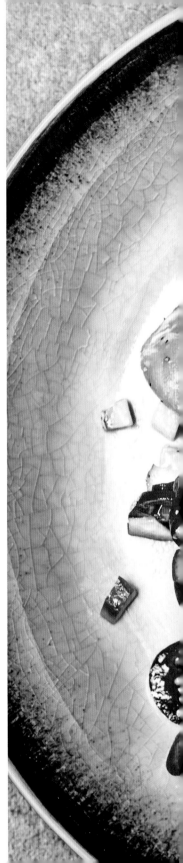

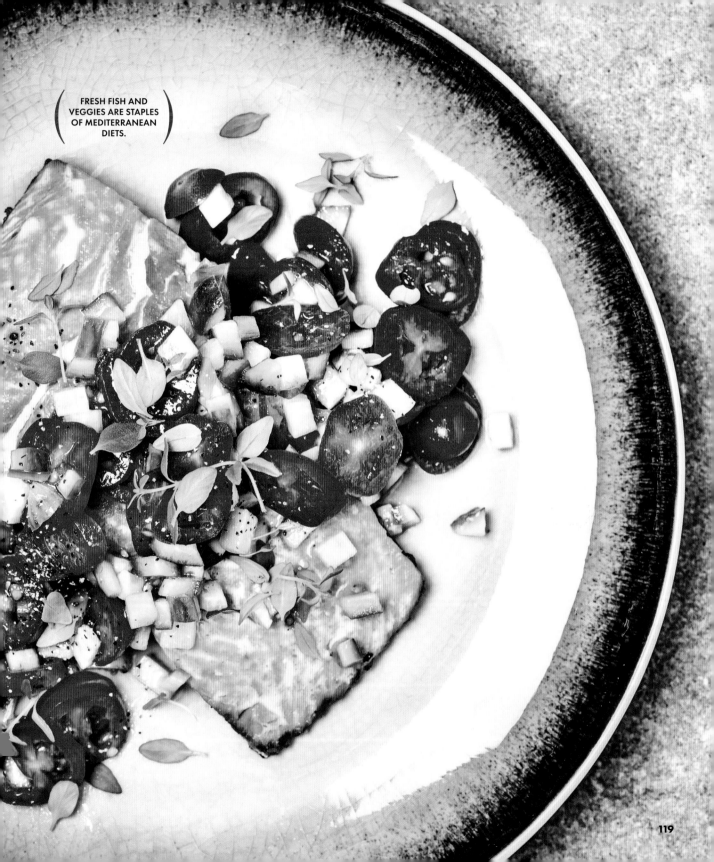

FRESH FISH AND VEGGIES ARE STAPLES OF MEDITERRANEAN DIETS.

The MIND Diet

Reduced risk of age-related memory loss, better heart health and a slimmer waistline are just some of the benefits of this eating plan.

What Is It?

As you can probably guess from the name, getting your brain in shape through food is what The MIND Diet (which stands for Mediterranean-DASH Intervention for Neurodegenerative Delay) is all about. With a focus on consuming foods that boost brain health and fight heart disease, it's a way of eating that fuses theories of both the Mediterranean and DASH diets, says Monica Auslander Moreno, M.S., R.D.N. Research shows it may help cut the risk for Alzheimer's and age-related memory and cognitive decline, but followers also experience weight loss and numerous health benefits, including cancer prevention. The MIND Diet has a stricter set of standards but can also be eaten intuitively. It's OK to veer off-course occasionally, says Moreno.

How It Works

The idea behind The MIND Diet is to promote positive neurological and cardiovascular outcomes by eating an anti-inflammatory diet, Moreno explains. By reducing inflammation, we may be able to prevent neurodegeneration and cardiovascular disease, as well as other inflammatory conditions. One study found those who adhered to The MIND Diet had a 53 percent lower risk of Alzheimer's disease.

What You'll Eat

With many brain-boosting foods suggested, a typical day of eating for MIND dieters can be satisfying, colorful and delicious. It includes plenty of small, wild, fatty fish; unsalted nuts, seeds and nut butters; at least seven servings of nonstarchy vegetables per day; legumes; fruit; dairy, like yogurt and kefir; whole unprocessed grains; and other healthy fats, like olive oil and avocados. A serving of red wine is considered appropriate.

Foods to Avoid

Steer clear of processed, refined grains, like most cereals, white bread or white flour products, and white rice; hydrogenated oils; fatty or processed meats; sugared dairy; candies and large amounts of added salt; fast food; butter or margarine; excessive cheese; and excessive red meat, suggests Moreno. "These foods—and processed meats, charred meats and certain chemicals and additives—can cause inflammatory changes that can contribute to the damage of cells and, in particular, brain cells."

THE PROS

- Laying off processed, sugary, salty and fried foods will definitely boost overall health and reduce the risk of certain diseases that would normally be caused by inflammation. Avoiding these foods will also lead to weight loss, especially if you stick to consuming 1,200 to 1,500 calories a day.

- This diet is easy to follow, since there are fewer restrictions than with many other eating plans.

THE CONS

- "Anytime someone disrupts their routine, there is bound to be resistance and a potential binge/failure/anxiety cycle," says Monica Auslander Moreno, M.S., R.D.N. Set incremental and realistic goals, and budget for veering off the program at times, all while incorporating healthy lifestyle changes.

- The higher-quality foods required to follow this program can become a pricier option.

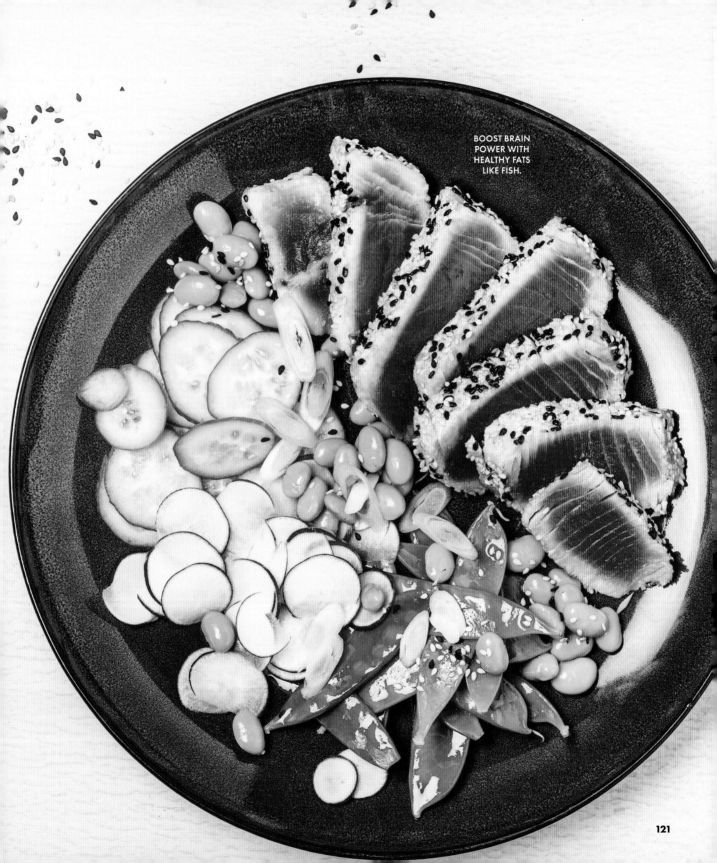

BOOST BRAIN
POWER WITH
HEALTHY FATS
LIKE FISH.

Noom

This weight-loss app prioritizes behavioral changes, virtual coaching and a "stoplight" food-labeling approach to promote lasting results.

What Is It?

Founded in 2008, Noom is a weight-loss app that allows you to track exercise, food and body weight, and connects you to a nutrition and exercise coach who will help personalize your plan.

Although nutrition and exercise are key components of the program, Noom approaches weight loss and wellness from a bigger perspective, says Meghan Wood, director of coaching operations at Noom.

"Our plans are designed around skill-building and measurable goal-setting. We don't help you just identify your goals, but also why they are your goals and the actions it'll take to get to those goals," she says.

How It Works

Noom doesn't prescribe a specific diet plan—rather, it's a behavior-change program that aims to help you better understand the content and value of the foods you're eating. Noom does this by labeling foods as red, yellow or green, depending on their caloric density, and giving you a daily budget for each. The red label is for foods with high-caloric density; yellow is for foods that should be consumed in moderation; and green is for foods low in caloric density, meaning you can eat them in large amounts.

Every user is also matched with a personal health coach and encouraged to connect with other users for support.

Preliminary research backs up the diet's effectiveness: A study published in the journal *Scientific Reports* found that about 78 percent of Noom users reported losing weight if they used the app for at least six months.

What You'll Eat

Green foods include fruits and vegetables, plus whole grains, nonfat dairy, potatoes, tofu, egg whites and coffee. Yellow foods include lean meats; low-fat dairy; processed grains; and nutritious but calorie-dense foods like salmon, avocado and quinoa. Focus on these foods first before sprinkling in the "red" options.

Foods to Avoid

"Red doesn't mean 'never,'" says Wood, just "in moderation." Red foods include choices like hamburgers, French fries, pizza, cake and potato chips, for example. Also labeled red: high-fat animal products and nut butters.

THE PROS

- Because Noom is focused on behavior change, it may lead to better results and lifestyle changes in the long-term.

- "I'm drawn to the encouragement of an all-foods-can-fit style of eating," says dietitian Elizabeth Shaw, M.S., R.D.N., owner of Shaw Simple Swap.

- Research shows that both internet-based social support and food tracking tools can improve weight-loss success.

THE CONS

- Noom will cost anywhere from $17 to $59 per month, depending on how far ahead you pay.

- While the stoplight food-labeling approach can make food choices easier, it can also be problematic. "I fear [the user] will label foods as 'good' and 'bad,'" says Shaw.

- "Most clients who come to me are looking for a detailed plan and direction," says Shaw. This app doesn't provide that.

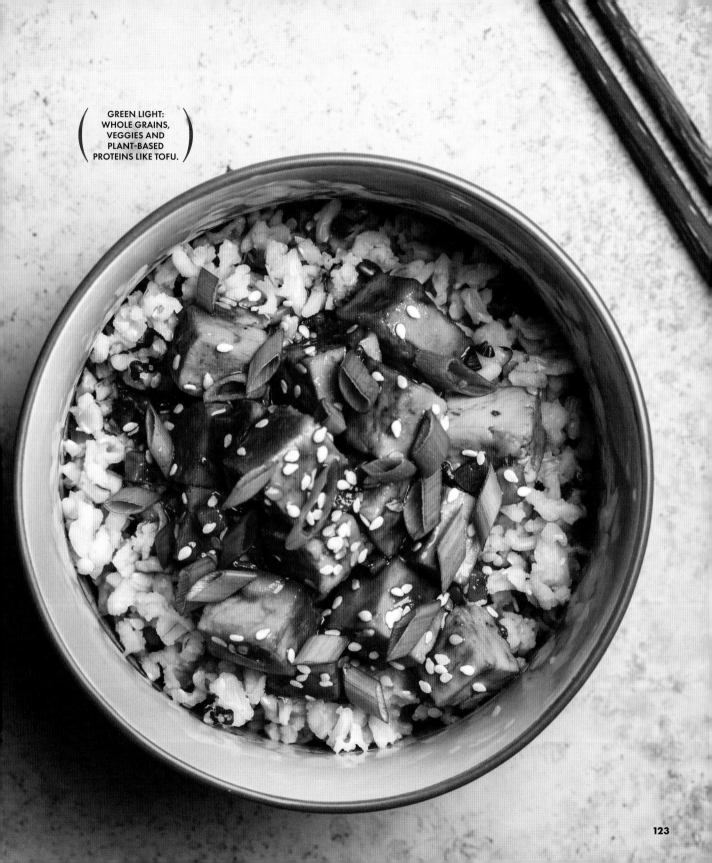

GREEN LIGHT: WHOLE GRAINS, VEGGIES AND PLANT-BASED PROTEINS LIKE TOFU.

The Paleo Diet

This low-carb weight-loss plan will help you lose weight, but it might not be sustainable for everyone.

What Is It?

This meat-lovers' diet plan has been trendy for more than a decade, thanks to Loren Cordain, Ph.D., who penned *The Paleo Diet* in 2002 (updated in 2010). Its premise is that you should eat the way our Paleolithic-era ancestors did 10,000 years ago. On this high-protein diet, you'll eliminate packaged foods, legumes and grains while emphasizing foods you'd find as a hunter or gatherer—meats, fresh vegetables, fruits and eggs.

How It Works

You'll probably need to overhaul the food in your kitchen and pantry, because a lot of what you've been eating on a Western diet isn't allowed. Paleo advocates believe that modern agricultural practices and manufacturing processes have created foods that are damaging our bodies. Wheat, especially, is linked to inflammation on this plan—so you'll need to cut it out and get your fiber from fruits and veggies instead. You'll probably lose weight if you were already eating a poor diet high in processed foods (particularly carbohydrates), fast foods, pizza and junk food before embarking on Paleo.

What You'll Eat

If you like the idea of loading up your plate with a large portion of meat and not having to bother counting fat, calories or portion sizes, you may enjoy Paleo. You can eat pasture-raised or grass-fed beef, lamb, pork, poultry and organ meats. Wild-caught fish are recommended, as well as raw nuts, healthy fats, and fruits and vegetables.

Foods to Avoid

Ditch all processed foods, added sugar and/or high-fructose corn syrup, artificial sweeteners, grains (including pasta, bread and rice), corn, legumes and peanut butter. Wine and beer are also considered off-limits, but some gluten-free spirits and low-sugar hard ciders are allowed.

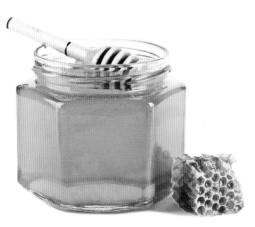

THE PROS

- Cleaning up your diet by eliminating processed carbs, sugar and junk food will likely result in weight loss, and can reduce inflammation and improve blood sugar levels.

- "Most clients I work with who follow a Paleo pattern find themselves eating more fruits and vegetables and become more intentional with their eating," says health coach Meghan Lyle, R.D.N.

THE CONS

- Some people use this as a license to eat red meat every day. Not only is this completely different from how our ancestors would have subsisted, but it's also not advisable if you want to reduce your risk of heart disease, diabetes, dementia or cancer, says Lyle.

- If you're already consuming a balanced diet that's low in processed foods and high in fruits, vegetables, lean proteins, whole grains, low-fat dairy and nuts and seeds, the likelihood of seeing significant weight loss with Paleo will be less, says Lyle.

- A Paleo Diet can be expensive, since it relies heavily on more expensive meats and fish.

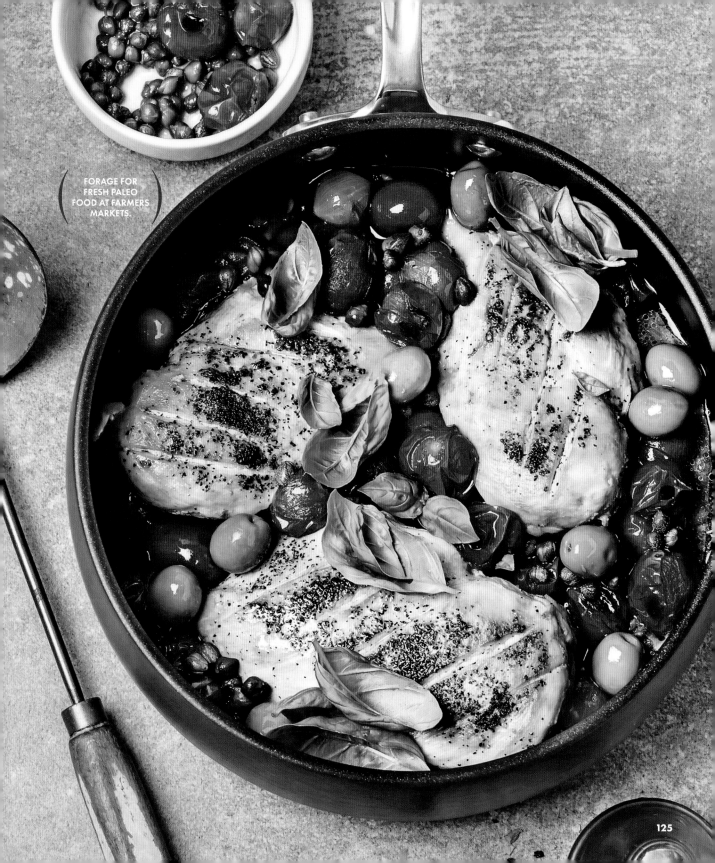

FORAGE FOR FRESH PALEO FOOD AT FARMERS MARKETS.

125

The Plant Paradox Diet

This controversial diet calls for cutting foods containing lectins, a protein found in plants, in order to reduce inflammation in the body.

What Is It?

The Plant Paradox diet book was published by former cardiac surgeon Steven Gundry, M.D., in April 2017. It gained attention when singer Kelly Clarkson credited the diet for helping her lose 37 pounds and manage a thyroid condition. Gundry designed the diet based on the idea that lectins (a plant protein found in many foods) are toxic and cause inflammation in the body. "While I believe that plants should be the cornerstone of a healthy diet, some plants clearly don't want you to eat them and will make you pay for it—hence the 'plant paradox,'" says Gundry.

How It Works

Scientists believe the lectin proteins were originally intended as a defense mechanism for plants to prevent them from being eaten. That's why they set off an adverse reaction in the human body. "Lectins...create a leaky gut, inflammation, brain fog, arthritis, autoimmune disease and heart disease," writes Gundry.

After studying his own patients, Gundry found a limited-lectin diet created in improvements in biomarkers for inflammation. He believes a lectin-free diet can help prevent weight gain and boost health.

What You'll Eat

The Plant Paradox allows cruciferous vegetables like cauliflower and broccoli, leafy greens like lettuce and spinach, root vegetables like carrots, herbs, limited dairy, fish, seafood and small amounts of pasture-raised poultry and meat, as well as certain plant proteins. Also on the menu are resistant starches (sweet potatoes and green bananas); nonwheat flours; small amounts of certain nuts and seeds (walnuts, pecans, flaxseeds, among others); avocado; and chocolate that contains 72 percent cacao or more.

Foods to Avoid

Refined starches (pasta, potatoes, rice, bread); most fruits; certain vegetables (tomatoes and cucumbers unless peeled and deseeded, peppers, zucchini, squash); all grains and legumes; grain- or soybean-fed animal products and cashews, peanuts and chia and pumpkin seeds.

THE PROS

- "The encouragement of fewer processed, high-sugar foods is a benefit," says Elizabeth Shaw, M.S., R.D.N., owner of Shaw Simple Swaps.

- Even those who have been eating clean lose weight when they try this diet, says Gundry.

THE CONS

- "Any diet that restricts healthy plant foods should be scrutinized carefully," says Julieanna Hever, M.S., R.D.

- "The claim that lectins are harmful creates a false sense of fear," says Shaw. A review in the *Journal of Cereal Science* found that lectins don't actually have a negative effect on your health.

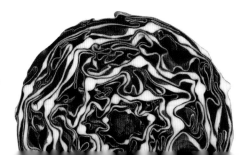

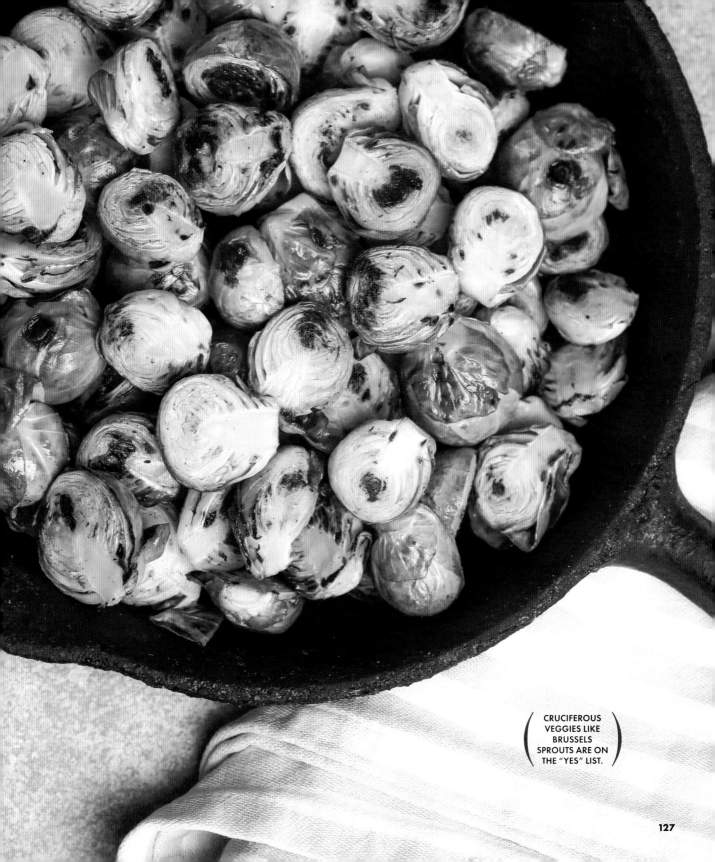

CRUCIFEROUS VEGGIES LIKE BRUSSELS SPROUTS ARE ON THE "YES" LIST.

Portion Control Diet

If dieting isn't your thing, this non-diet—which requires limiting the portions of any food you select—may be right for you.

What Is It?

What if you were told that you could follow a diet that consisted of any and all the foods you love, with the only limitation being the amount of this food you can have during a single sitting? Would you sign up? This plan, known as the portion control diet, is based on the idea that portion control is the ultimate key to weight loss.

There are several interpretations of this way of eating, with different books on the marketplace from various authors. Some simply recommend easy-to-measure serving sizes; others focus on creating nutritious meals and stopping when you're full; and some require tracking every calorie you eat to make sure you don't go over a recommended daily allotment of calories.

Sounds tempting, right? One thing is for certain—it's an effective long-term weight-loss solution for those who have the willpower to measure out their portions, stop when they're done eating that amount, and fully commit.

This concept is, in its purest sense, a good one, agrees Christen Cupples Cooper, Ed.D., R.D.N., assistant professor and founding director of the Nutrition and Dietetics Program at the College of Health Professions at Pace University in New York City. "Essentially, it promotes intuitive eating, which is listening to our bodies and eating the amount of food that we are hungry for—not more and not less," she explains. "This worked well for millennia, before our senses of hunger and fullness became distorted by the 24/7 availability of junk food," adds Cooper.

For those who can fight the urge to finish a giant, juicy burger, or can enjoy a small portion of pizza instead of devouring two slices, this diet can be effective.

How It Works

In its simplest form, the portion control diet works by allowing you to eat any food on the menu or at the grocery store, with the sole limitation being the portion size.

Your caloric allotment may differ from the next person; however, it's typically based on BMI, or body mass index, as well as your level of activity. "The body naturally burns about 2,000 calories per day just to maintain its normal functions,

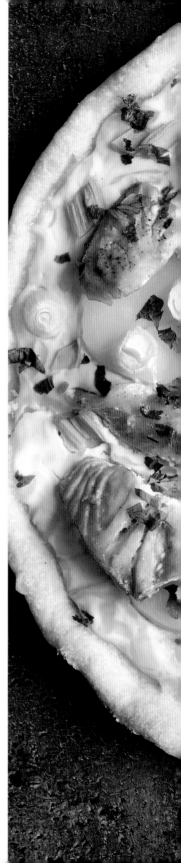

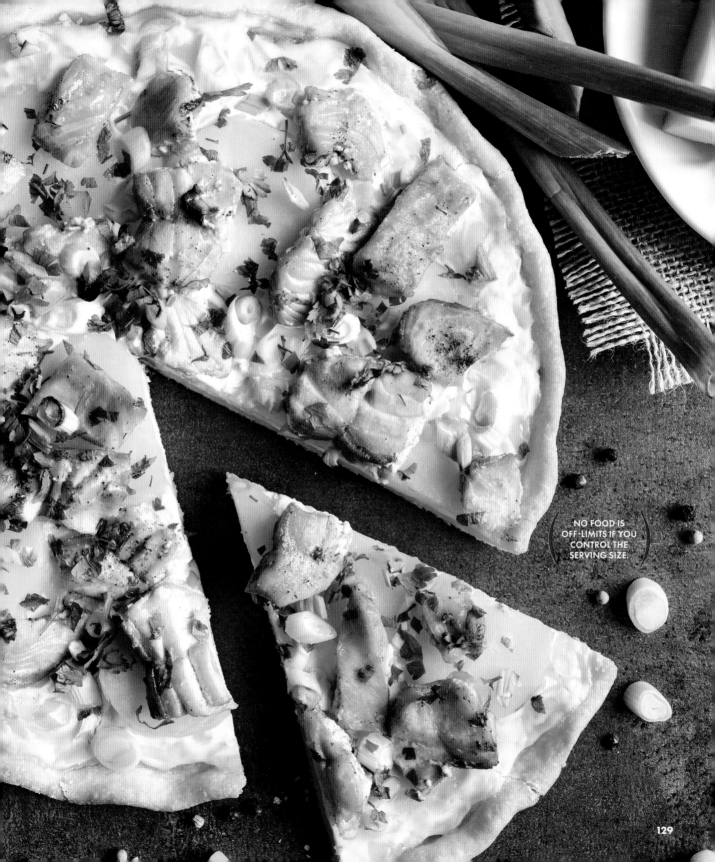

NO FOOD IS OFF-LIMITS IF YOU CONTROL THE SERVING SIZE.

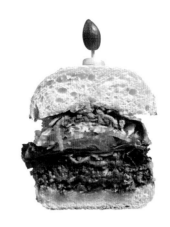

but this way of eating recommends that you eat under 2,000 calories per day to create a deficit," explains Lisa Samuels, R.D., founder of The Happie House in New York. Eating plans that contain 1,200 to 1,500 calories daily will help most women lose weight safely. Plans with 1,500 to 1,800 calories each day are suitable for men and for women who weigh more or who exercise regularly, according to the National Heart, Lung, and Blood Institute.

If you were following a portion control plan, like The Ultimate Volumetrics Diet created by Barbara Rolls, Ph.D., professor of nutritional sciences and obesity researcher at Penn State, you would focus on eating high-volume foods that fill you up (like fruits, veggies and broth-based soups) and not have to worry about counting calories.

What You'll Eat

The entire point of following a portion control diet is that you don't have to give up your favorite foods—simply control portion sizes and overall caloric intake to an amount that allows you to keep your appetite-regulating hormone, leptin, at bay so that you don't feel hungry.

"The goal is to eat foods that contain enough fat, protein and fiber to make you feel full and satiated longer," explains Carolyn Dean, M.D., N.D., medical advisory board member at Nutritional Magnesium Association. Eat your favorite foods mixed in with good fats such as avocado, nuts and seeds; a moderate amount of protein; and fiber from vegetables such as cauliflower,

cabbage, garden cress, bok choy, broccoli and Brussels sprouts, as well as whole grains, Dean says. The protein sources she recommends include wild-caught salmon and other wild-caught fish, grass-fed organic beef, grass-fed buffalo/bison meat, organic free-range chicken, lamb and beef (nuts, beans and legumes for vegetarians).

This combination will help you feel fuller longer while keeping calories at around 300 for breakfast, 400 for lunch, 500 for dinner and 125 for each of two snacks if you're on a 1,500-calorie plan, according to Dean.

As long as you stay in the parameters of your daily calorie allotment, even if you give in to that slice of chocolate cake or extra scoop of ice cream, and participate in moderate exercise, you will lose weight and be able to stay on this plan without giving up your favorite foods or starving yourself.

Foods to Avoid

There are no food groups or food items that are eliminated from this diet, which is its main attraction. Stick to your calorie recommendations and weight loss will ensue.

THE PROS

- You don't have to eliminate foods, which not only makes it easier to follow, but more enjoyable than diets that cut out certain food groups. There is also an emphasis on eating enough food so you don't feel ravenous.

- "You will lose weight on a portion control diet if you are able to burn more calories than you consume," says Carolyn Dean, M.D., N.D. Since you won't feel deprived, you can be emotionally satisfied to eat smaller portions of them.

THE CONS

- The diet doesn't teach healthy eating. "Some people might use it as an excuse to eat unhealthy options every day, so long as they stay within their calorie limit," says Lisa Samuels, R.D.

- Counting calories requires a great deal of commitment, so this might not be the most ideal plan for someone with a busy schedule that requires them to travel frequently and dine out at restaurants, where it is undoubtedly more difficult to control portions.

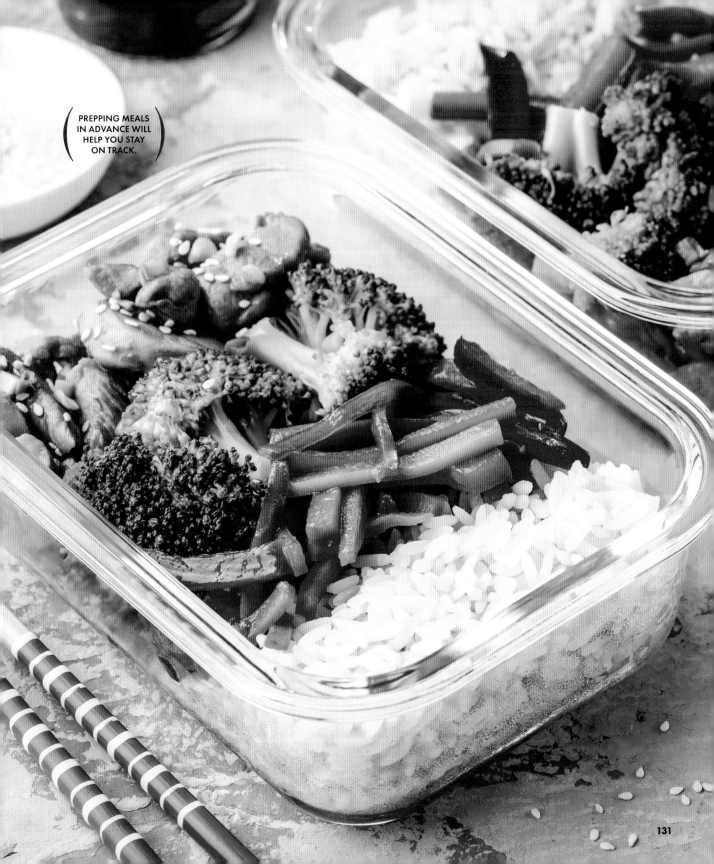

PREPPING MEALS IN ADVANCE WILL HELP YOU STAY ON TRACK.

Raw Food Diet

This diet has a popular social media following, but are you really ready to eat (mostly) cold food for the rest of your life?

What Is It?

Before we learned how to utilize fire to heat up food, we ate everything raw—meat, vegetables, fruits, etc. While we didn't have a choice back then, people today still follow this type of eating religiously. Just as its name suggests, the raw food diet revolves around the concept of eating primarily uncooked vegetables, fruits, nuts, seeds and sprouted grains.

How It Works

The premise is that heating food lowers its nutrient content and makes it harder to digest, so fewer vitamins, minerals and enzymes get into the body. But while cooking some foods may indeed lower their nutritional value, many times, cooking actually makes food easier for the body to digest and absorb nutrients, explains Roger E. Adams, Ph.D., a Houston-based dietitian. "Purists believe cooking food kills its nutritional value and may actually make food toxic or harmful to the body," he says. "Additionally, claims are being made that a raw food diet will clear up headaches, alleviate arthritis and boost your memory."

But while eating more fruits and vegetables will improve your health, there is scant evidence that cooking foods is actually harmful or toxic.

What You'll Eat

Organizationally, this diet is relatively easy to follow—it just includes foods that are uncooked and unprocessed, which essentially leaves only raw fruits and vegetables, raw nuts and seeds, sprouted grains, and, for some, raw meats, eggs, seafoods and unpasteurized dairy products. Cold-pressed oils, such as olive oil and coconut oil, fall into the category of "raw" because they're made without heat-processing techniques.

Foods to Avoid

Any food heated above 118 degrees Fahrenheit. This temperature cutoff is set because most enzymes are deactivated above this temperature. However, the acidic environment of the stomach destroys most enzymes anyway, so not cooking to preserve enzymes is usually a moot point, says Adams. There isn't really a food you can adequately cook at 118 degrees, so you can warm up your food to this temperature without supposedly altering the enzymes. You could warm nuts, seeds, soups and teas to improve palatability, mouthfeel and provide a warm bite, he adds.

While cooking isn't part of the protocol, other techniques, like blending, juicing, sprouting and dehydrating, are acceptable.

THE PROS

- If you want to follow a vegan diet, then this is definitely one for you. "You can make the raw food diet meet a vegan lifestyle," Adams explains. "If you are gluten intolerant or gluten sensitive, a raw food diet may be a good option, since most of the raw foods on this diet are naturally free of gluten."

- You'll eliminate highly processed foods, which has health benefits.

- You'll probably lose weight. The diet is rich in high-fiber fruits and veggies, which makes them very filling, and you'll likely take in fewer calories.

THE CONS

- Eating raw meats, egg, seafood and dairy products can create a serious health risk, since harmful bacteria may be lurking in these foods.

- If you avoid raw meat, dairy and fish, you may be missing out on good protein sources, healthy fats like omega-3 fatty acids and nutrients like calcium, iron and vitamins D and B12. And avoiding beans and grains means you'll miss out on fiber.

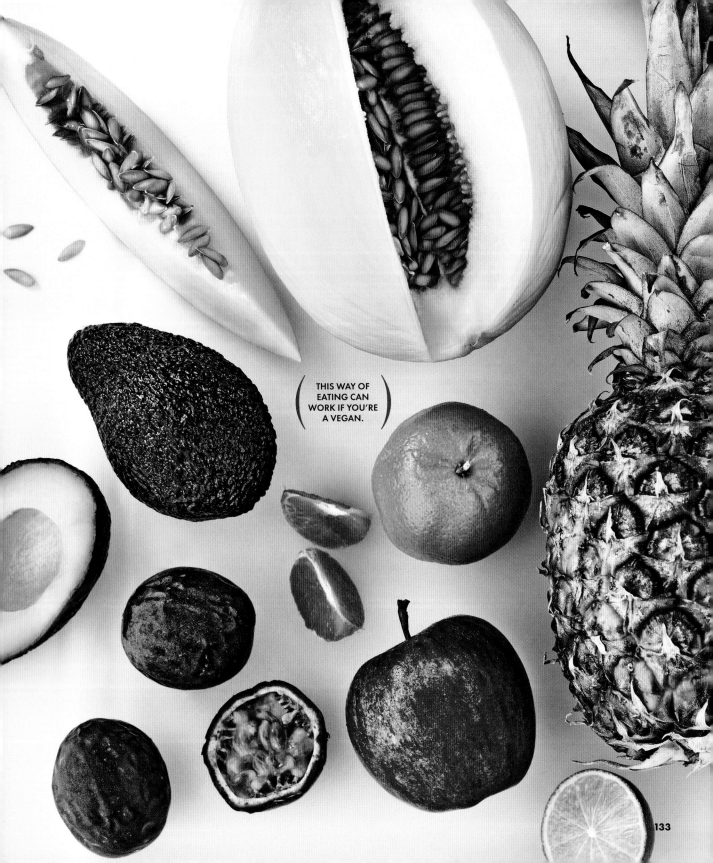

THIS WAY OF
EATING CAN
WORK IF YOU'RE
A VEGAN.

The Setpoint Diet

Unlike many of the diets trending today, this one takes a commonsense approach, and it's highly regarded by nutrition experts.

What Is It?

The Setpoint Diet focuses on a slow adjustment and is considered to be a lifestyle change that can be followed for the long haul.

In essence, The Setpoint Diet is a way of eating that is meant to help your body "reset" to a lower weight that it can maintain long-term. The theory is that humans are born with a genetically determined weight that the body will want to reach and lock into for life, and you can achieve this by getting back to your set point. "The strategy for The Setpoint Diet is a commonsense approach because it doesn't involve giving up entire food groups or fasting," explains Roger E. Adams, Ph.D., owner of eatrightfitness.com. "You'll eat whole, natural foods to help lower inflammation, restore healthy gut bacteria and balance hormones."

How It Works

Perhaps the trickiest part of following The Setpoint Diet is the fact that there is no set macronutrient or calorie requirement. "The diet works by focusing on stored body-fat levels and regulating your appetite and metabolism through your hormones, which is why it's more of a lifestyle approach than a 'diet,'" says Miriam Amselem, a holistic nutritionist. "An elevated set-point weight is usually due to eating heavily processed foods and sugar, [or suffering from] chronic stress and sleep deprivation, which elevate cortisol levels and affect weight gain."

By reducing consumption of high-calorie foods and processed carbohydrates, you would likely lower your total calorie count and lose weight, explains Christen Cupples Cooper, Ed.D., R.D.N.

What You'll Eat

To reach your set point, the diet recommends 10 servings of nonstarchy vegetables (like spinach, broccoli, cauliflower, asparagus or romaine lettuce) a day; plus three to five daily servings of nutrient-dense protein, such as salmon, egg whites, lean meat or nonfat Greek yogurt; three to six daily servings of fats from whole foods, such as flaxseeds, almonds, olive oil, coconut, olives and chia seeds; and up to three daily servings of low-sugar fruits.

Foods to Avoid

Stay away from sugary beverages and snacks, processed baked goods and breads. By avoiding those high-carb foods as well as limiting starchy vegetables and alcohol, you may reach your weight-loss goals faster.

THE PROS

- "Increasing your fiber intake helps to fill you up without filling you out, while consuming lean, quality proteins can have a great satiety effect, leading to fewer calories consumed by the end of the day," notes Roger E. Adams, Ph.D.

- "The focus on healthy gut bacteria is key—we are finding more and more research pointing to controls in the gut for weight loss and regulation," says Adams.

THE CONS

- The elimination of most grains and starchy foods will be difficult for many people, since these are staples in the American diet. Replacing these with nonstarchy veggies and whole foods with healthy fats can help you feel full.

- Dieters might get impatient, says nutritionist Miriam Amselem. "It's a slow system, so it's best for someone who's looking for an overall lifestyle change and not looking to 'diet.'"

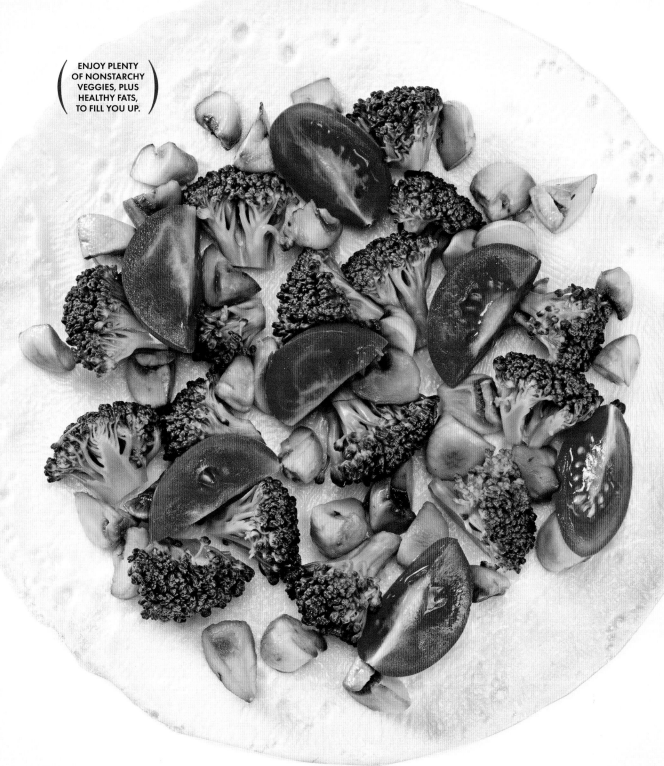

ENJOY PLENTY
OF NONSTARCHY
VEGGIES, PLUS
HEALTHY FATS,
TO FILL YOU UP.

The South Beach Diet

This heart-healthy, low-carb plan is one that you can stick to for life, if you enjoy the foods—and like eating six times a day!

What Is It?

The South Beach Diet has been around since the 1990s, when heart doctor Arthur Agatston, M.D., created the program. His book, *The South Beach Diet*, came out in 2003; both the book and diet have been through several iterations since then, but are still quite popular.

Today, you can follow the diet by having meals delivered to your door. There's no counting calories, fat grams, carbs or anything else, if you don't want to. Or you can buy the book and follow the diet rules on your own, buying and preparing your own food and keeping track of macros.

How It Works

The diet references the glycemic index (GI) of foods to help determine which carbs to avoid. It's based on research that shows low-GI carbs—like zucchini, cucumbers and greens—can help you drop pounds and keep blood sugar levels steady. Phase 1 is very low-carb, because research has shown that reducing carbs is one of the most effective strategies for helping to jump-start weight loss. Health experts like that this diet is flexible and includes most foods, says Sonya Angelone, M.S., R.D.N., spokesperson for the Academy of Nutrition and Dietetics.

What You'll Eat

You'll eat six times a day on every phase of this plan! In Phase 1, the focus is on lean proteins such as skinless poultry, seafood, lean beef and soy products. It also includes high-fiber vegetables; low-fat dairy products; and healthy, monounsaturated fats, like those in avocados, nuts and seeds. "It restricts foods that people often overeat," says Angelone. (Think chips, wine and desserts.) "This can give people the momentum to continue with the process." Phase 2 adds back some whole grains and more fruits and vegetables, which are higher in carbs—plus red wine! This flexibility allows dieters to adhere more easily to the plan, but you'll still need to monitor portions. Phase 3 is the maintenance phase, which requires almost 30 percent of calories to come from carbs (140 grams) on a 2,000-calorie diet. Exercising for 30 minutes a day is recommended.

Foods to Avoid

In Phase 1 you'll limit grains, including whole-grain breads, whole-wheat pasta, fruit and brown rice, says Angelone. After this initial period, these foods can be added back in limited portions—but overly processed foods are discouraged.

THE PROS

- This diet is restrictive for the first two weeks but then adds back healthy carbohydrates, which makes it both more nutritionally balanced and more flexible so it's easier to follow over time.

- There's a mindful-eating component that teaches you to slow down and enjoy your food, which can help you eat less.

THE CONS

- Overly restricting carbs may cause headaches, mental and physical fatigue and dizziness, says Sonya Angelone, R.D.N.

- It's expensive, especially if you go for the delivery meal plan, which starts at $10.36/day and up. Even if you DIY, the high-quality food required on this plan can be costly.

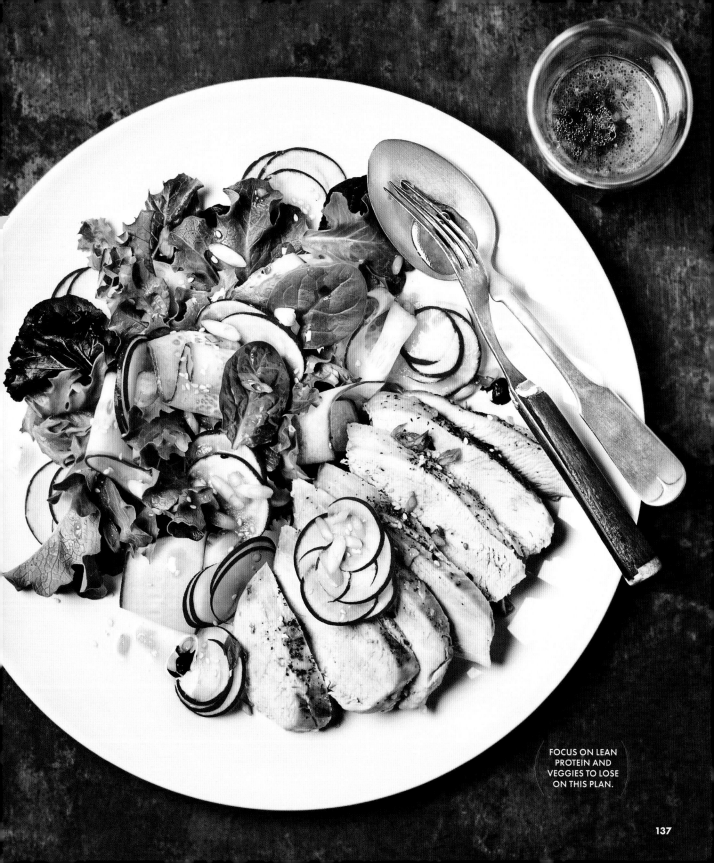

FOCUS ON LEAN PROTEIN AND VEGGIES TO LOSE ON THIS PLAN.

Therapeutic Lifestyle Changes Diet

Also known as the TLC diet, your doctor may have recommended this eating plan and lifestyle to lower cholesterol level.

What Is It?

Therapeutic Lifestyle Changes Diet is a three-part program that incorporates diet, physical activity and weight management. The National Heart, Lung, and Blood Institute designed it to help people lower high LDL ("bad") cholesterol, which increases the risk of heart disease.

How It Works

You can make improvements in your LDL cholesterol by doing the following: getting fewer than 7 percent of your daily calories from saturated fat; decreasing dietary cholesterol to less than 200 mg/day; adding 5 to 10 grams per day of soluble fiber; and adding 2 grams per day of plant stanols or sterols. By increasing daily exercise and aiming to lose even 10 pounds if you're overweight, you can reduce your LDL number.

What You'll Eat

You'll eat fruits, vegetables, whole grains, low-fat or nonfat dairy products, fish, skinless poultry, and, in moderate amounts, lean meats. You'll also try to eat 10 to 25 grams per day of soluble fiber. This type of fiber helps lower the risk of heart disease. Many plant foods are rich in soluble fiber, as are oat bran, barley, nuts, seeds, beans, lentils and peas. "When you're eating foods that contain cholesterol, soluble fiber will bind with the cholesterol so it's not absorbed," says NYC–based registered dietitian Lisa Stollman, M.A., R.D.N., author of *The Trim Traveler*. You should try to incorporate healthy fats, like those found in vegetable oils, most nuts, olives, avocados and fatty fish, such as salmon.

Foods to Avoid

You'll be reducing saturated fat, trans fat and cholesterol in your diet. Saturated fat is found in fatty cuts of meat, poultry with the skin, whole-milk dairy products, and some vegetable oils. Trans fats have largely been phased out today, but may still be found in some stick margarine, foods like French fries, and some baked goods.

This plan recommends followers eat two or fewer egg yolks per week, due to concerns about higher cholesterol levels, but that fear has since been disproven.

THE PROS

- The TLC diet calls itself a "no-deprivation plan." If you're enjoying a treat, look for those made with unsaturated oil, egg whites or egg substitutes, and fat-free milk.

- You're allowed to have alcohol, but keep it to one drink a day for women and two for men.

- You probably will lower your bad cholesterol number and reduce your heart disease risk. Getting regular exercise is great for your heart and your waistline, and it's a pillar of this plan.

THE CONS

- "I was somewhat surprised when I saw that the diet suggests only two egg yolks a week, because we've seen from various studies that eating eggs does not increase cholesterol," says Lisa Stollman, R.D.N. The worst components for cholesterol are saturated fat and trans fat, she says.

- Stollman says plant-based proteins should play a greater part in the plan. "We see the biggest change in cholesterol levels in people who eat plant-based meals," she notes.

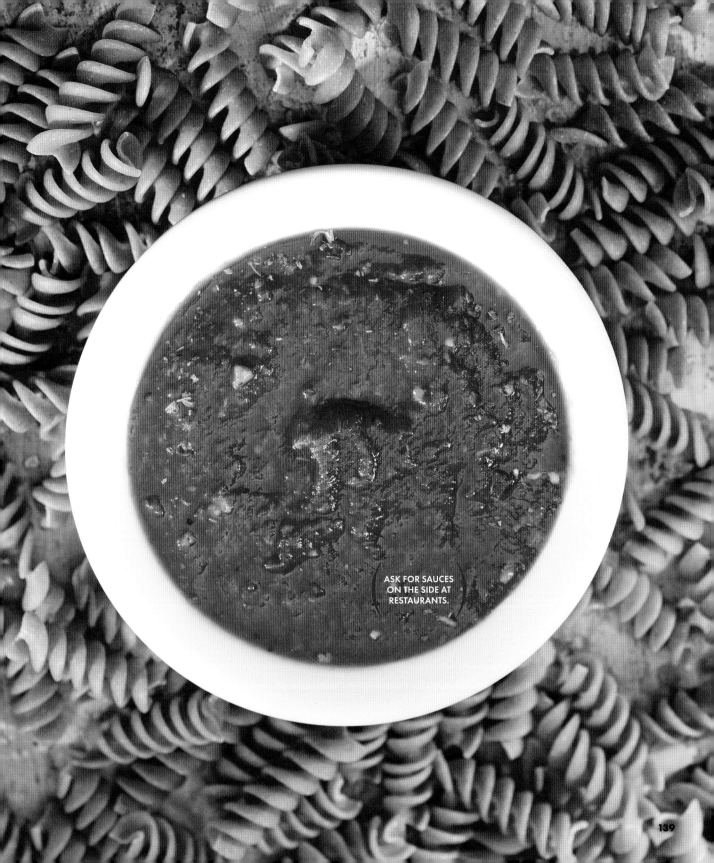

ASK FOR SAUCES ON THE SIDE AT RESTAURANTS.

Vegan/Vegetarian/ Plant-Based Diets

These veggie-heavy diets have proven health benefits that might convince you to cut back on meat and dairy consumption.

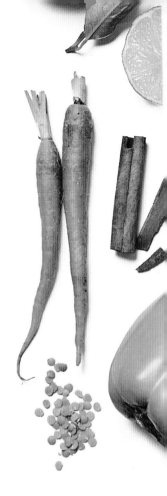

What Is It?

Vegetarian and vegan lifestyles aren't new—but they've been surging in popularity, thanks to documentaries like *The Game Changers* (2018) and celebrities like Beyoncé, who tout the health perks of plant-based eating. A 2017 Nielsen Homescan survey found that 39 percent of Americans are actively trying to eat more plant foods.

Vegetarianism is a general term for people who don't eat animal products, though lacto-vegetarians eat dairy; pescatarians eat fish and ovo-vegetarians eat eggs. Veganism means avoiding all food products derived from animals, including meat, eggs and dairy. All of these fall under the "plant-based diet" label, which is a looser umbrella term for diets heavy on plant-sourced foods and light on— or free of—animal products.

How It Works

By reducing (high-calorie) animal products and increasing (lower-calorie) plant foods, you're eating more nutritionally dense foods, which can help you fill up faster on fewer calories, so you'll lose weight without feeling hungry all the time. Research on plant-based diets shows they're remarkably effective for weight loss; improving cholesterol, blood pressure and blood sugar levels; reversing diabetes; and alleviating certain chronic pain syndromes, says Neal Barnard, M.D., author of *The Vegan Starter Kit*.

What You'll Eat

The only real rule is to eliminate animal products in your diet, but if your goal is to lose weight, you'll need to focus on whole, unprocessed foods and plenty of produce—not junk food like candy and chips. "Emphasize vegetables, fruits, whole grains, legumes, mushrooms, nuts, seeds, herbs and spices for a well-rounded, nutritious diet and to achieve all the benefits associated with plant-based eating," says Julieanna Hever, M.S., R.D., C.P.T., author of *The Complete Idiot's Guide to Plant-Based Nutrition*.

Though the issue of adequate protein intake often comes up around vegan and vegetarian diets,

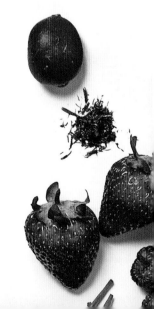

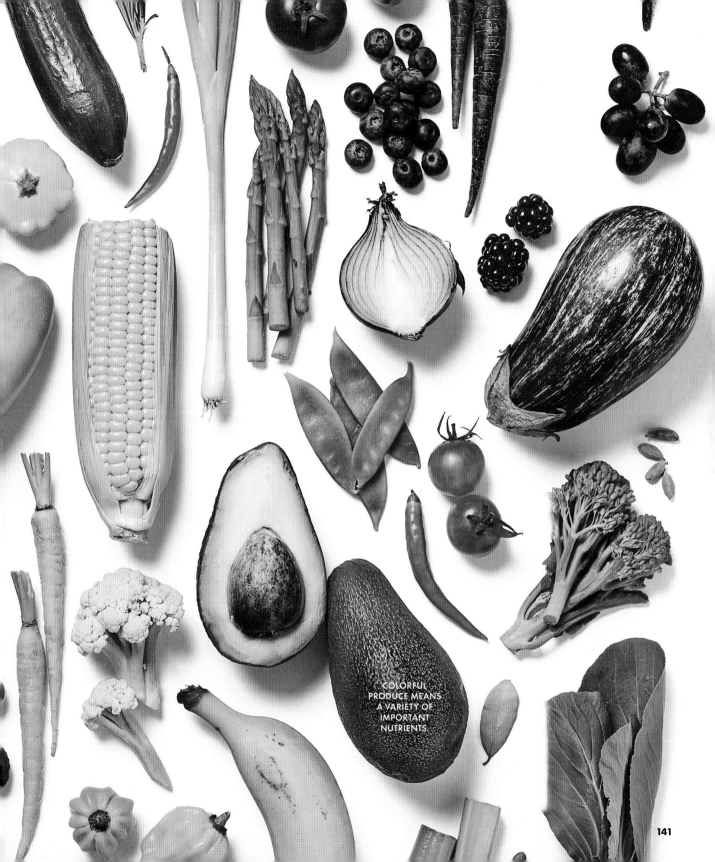

COLORFUL
PRODUCE MEANS
A VARIETY OF
IMPORTANT
NUTRIENTS

it's not actually a problem, says Barnard. Female vegans who want to consume the recommended 46 grams of protein daily could get an adequate amount by eating soy yogurt with almonds, nut butter on whole-wheat toast, cooked lentils and tofu, as well as broccoli, edamame and other veggies.

Foods to Avoid

Plant-based diets don't really have hard-and-fast rules, but you do need to keep in mind that they're not all equally healthy. Plenty of unhealthy processed foods are technically vegetarian or vegan (looking at you, white pasta, potato chips and some candy!) Plus, there's a growing selection of processed, plant-based alternatives to traditional meat and dairy products that don't exactly get nutritional gold stars, either.

"The risk of eating a plant-based diet is the inclusion of highly refined foods, since there's now an influx of commercial products available," says Hever. Faux-meat products may be able to help you transition to a plant-based life, but whole foods themselves are the better nutritional choice. If you want to lose weight, try to eliminate junk food. "[Ditch] items that contain added refined sugars, oils, flours and salts," Hever adds.

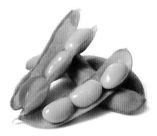

THE PROS

• There's a good chance that going plant-based will help you lose weight, especially if you reduce your fat intake.

• It may boost metabolism. "After a meal, your metabolism usually rises because you're absorbing nutrients. But after a person has been vegan for three months, their metabolism rises about 16 percent higher after a meal than before they were vegan," says Neal Barnard, M.D.,citing a study published in *The American Journal of Medicine.*

THE CONS

• When you eliminate food groups, you put yourself at risk for some nutrient deficiencies—namely iron, zinc, calcium, vitamins D and B12 and omega-3 fats, says Dawn Jackson Blatner, L.D.N. However, you can get all these nutrients from plant-based sources— except vitamin B12.

• You can still get vitamin B12 but it might come in a pill: "It's in a lot of fortified foods, like soy milk," says Barnard. "But I encourage most people to take a supplement regardless of their diet."

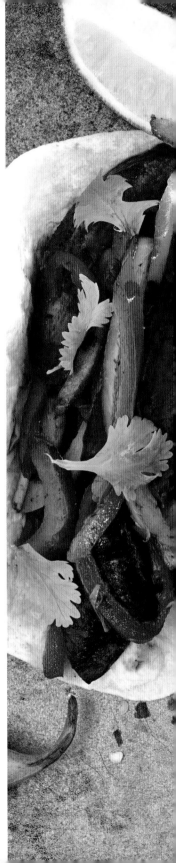

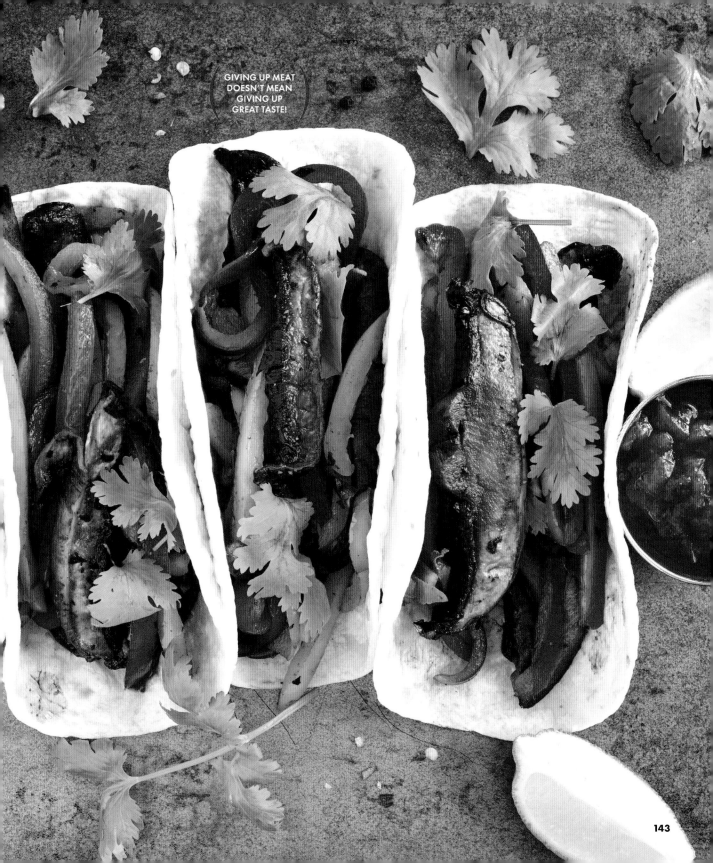

GIVING UP MEAT
DOESN'T MEAN
GIVING UP
GREAT TASTE!

The Whole30 Program

The elimination-style plan is designed to help you determine what foods might be affecting your health.

What Is It?

The Whole30 Program is an elimination diet of sorts, designed to help followers eat nutritious, whole foods (meaning foods in their original state or as close to it as possible) while cutting out certain food groups—particularly sugar, grains, dairy and legumes.

These foods are said to impact skin, weight, inflammation, digestive issues, allergies and energy, according to Whole30 co-creator Melissa Hartwig, a certified sports nutritionist, in the Whole30 book and website. That's why the diet instructs followers to strip those foods completely from their diet for one month. Doing this is promised to "change your life."

How It Works

Once you eliminate these foods from your diet, your body will "reset" (the diet claims), your cravings will be gone, your tastes will change and you will feel better, according to the Whole30 website.

After completing the 30 days, you can reintroduce foods back into your diet one at a time, whether that's sugar, dairy, grains or legumes. The founder suggests that if you don't miss a food and don't want to add it back in, you don't need to.

What You'll Eat

Lots of veggies. But you'll also eat "moderate portions" of meat, seafood and eggs; all fruit is allowed; plenty of natural fats (clarified butter, ghee, coconut oil, avocado, seeds) and herbs, spices and seasonings. You can have coffee and tea (hooray!), sparkling water, plain water, coconut water, vegetable juices, fruit juice—and kombucha as well. But no alcohol is allowed on the plan.

Foods to Avoid

For 30 days, you'll avoid: sugar in any form (real and artificial), alcohol, legumes, grains, tofu, any baked foods or junk foods (even if you think they're healthy), dairy, as well as any foods that contain carrageenan, MSG or sulfites.

Another thing you'll eliminate for a month? Weighing yourself.

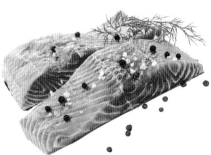

THE PROS

- "I like the program's focus on using lean proteins and plenty of fruits and vegetables," says Jessica Crandall Snyder, R.D., C.D.E., C.P.T.

- Those who like to be told just what they can and can't eat, rather than counting calories or tracking grams, may enjoy its specificity.

THE CONS

- Many health experts dislike the elimination portion of this plan—in particular, whole grains, beans and dairy. "Whole grains and beans are a significant source of fiber in the American diet, which we know we're already not getting enough of," says Crandall Snyder. Whole grains are important when it comes to decreasing LDL (bad) cholesterol, she says.

- Dairy is a great source of bone-boosting calcium and vitamin D—so don't stay off it too long, says Crandall Snyder.

- While you might lose weight, that's not the main point of this plan. So if you're looking for a quick fix and fast results, Whole30 probably isn't your top choice.

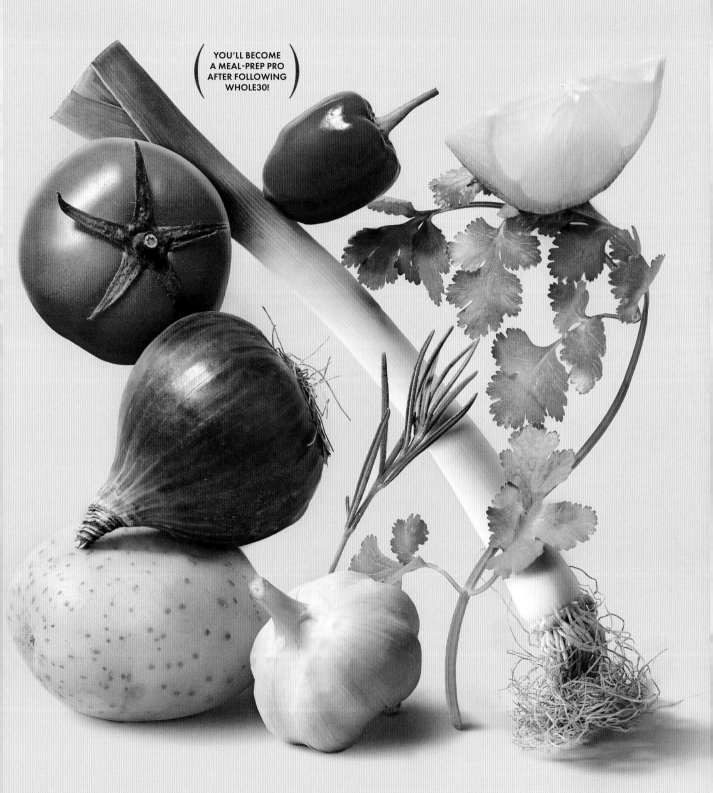

YOU'LL BECOME
A MEAL-PREP PRO
AFTER FOLLOWING
WHOLE30!

WW

Once known as Weight Watchers, the decades-old plan recently underwent a makeover and is now more nutritionally sound than ever.

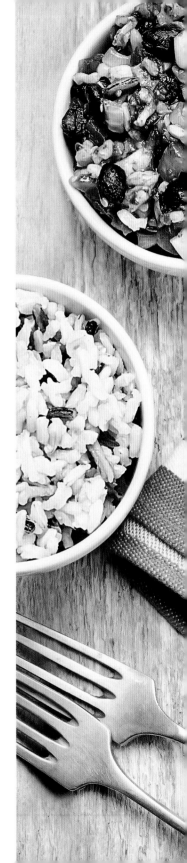

What Is It?

We're pretty sure you've heard of Weight Watchers (recently rebranded as WW). Maybe you've tried it, your mom did, or *someone* in your circle has counted points and attended Weight Watchers meetings.

The Weight Watchers plan started in the 1960s when founder Jean Nidetch invited friends into her Queens, New York, home once a week to discuss ideas on how to lose weight. Since then, millions of women and men globally have tried the Weight Watchers program. Many went to weekly meetings for a few decades until the online-only program of Weight Watchers Online was created in the early 2000s—geared toward members who didn't have access to in-person meetings or who didn't want this type of group support.

The Weight Watchers Freestyle program, launched in December 2017, encourages people to eat more fruits, vegetables and lean proteins, less sugar—and to avoid unhealthy fats as much as possible. They created a list of 200-plus foods that are ZeroPoint. This means members don't have to weigh, track and measure their consumption of these foods. They have to track the rest of the foods they eat by looking up the value Weight Watchers assigned them, and either writing them down or using the online app. Each member has a unique Daily SmartPoints Budget based on age, weight, activity level and gender. That number changes as their weight decreases.

How It Works

Weight Watchers allows members to eat any foods they want—nothing is off-limits. They also try to educate members on healthy habits, like practicing portion control for foods that aren't on their ZeroPoint list, learning moderation, and identifying some foods as healthier than others—like lean proteins, fruits and vegetables.

The lifestyle program encourages members to incorporate exercise—called "Activity"—into their routine while losing weight, earning FitPoints for cardio, strength and everyday activities like cleaning.

What You'll Eat

"The folks at Weight Watchers are constantly innovating the program, and the new program brings about a nice change to focus on not only the importance of fruits and vegetables

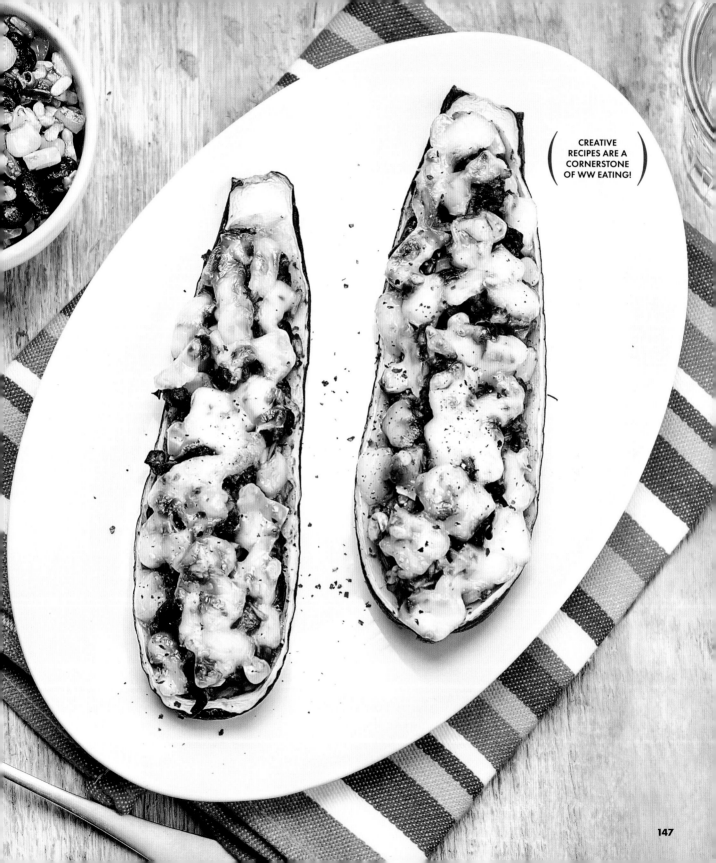

CREATIVE RECIPES ARE A CORNERSTONE OF WW EATING!

but also the importance of eating quality proteins," says Amy Gorin, M.S., R.D.N, owner of Amy Gorin Nutrition in the New York City area.

You can eat any foods you'd like, but Weight Watchers suggests you fill up on their ZeroPoint foods and round out your meals with healthy fats, whole grains and other foods you love. Some of the ZeroPoint foods include fish, skinless turkey breast, skinless chicken breast, vegetables, fruits, eggs, beans, tofu, nonfat unsweetened yogurt and lentils, to name a few. There is no portion limit to these foods, but the plan encourages members to eat until they're satisfied, not stuffed.

You'll weigh yourself weekly—which studies have shown is part of a habit that long-term successful dieters use—and then adjust your daily food budget accordingly.

Foods to Avoid

Members are encouraged to limit added sugars and unhealthy fats, like trans fats.

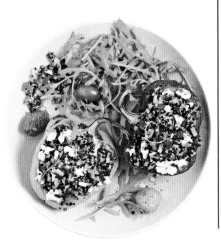

THE PROS

• WW has a popular service where you can get help from a trained coach online, 24/7.

• The plan encourages regular exercise where you aim to complete weekly fitness goals.

• "WW does a great job at steering people away from unhealthy choices," says Courtney Anaya, L.D.N. "Giving a higher SmartPoints value to pizza, alcohol and cake motivates a dieter to use his or her points wisely."

• There's a lot of inherent flexibility. "WW offers tools to create good habits," says Anaya.

THE CONS

• You'll pay weekly or monthly until you reach your goal weight and achieve Lifetime membership status.

• Weekly weigh-ins are required for members who attend "workshops"—and for some this can be uncomfortable. But only the person weighing you will see your results.

• If you're looking for superfast results, know that this program is designed for slower and steadier weight loss.

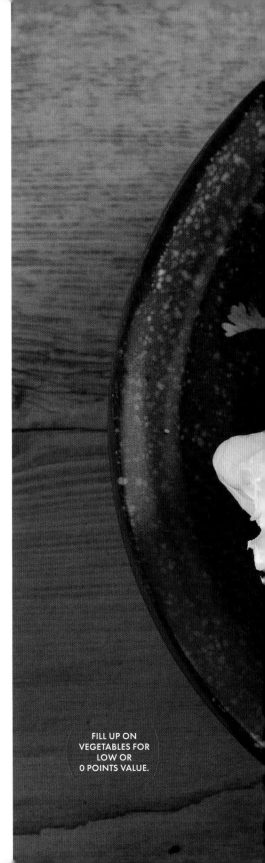

FILL UP ON VEGETABLES FOR LOW OR 0 POINTS VALUE.

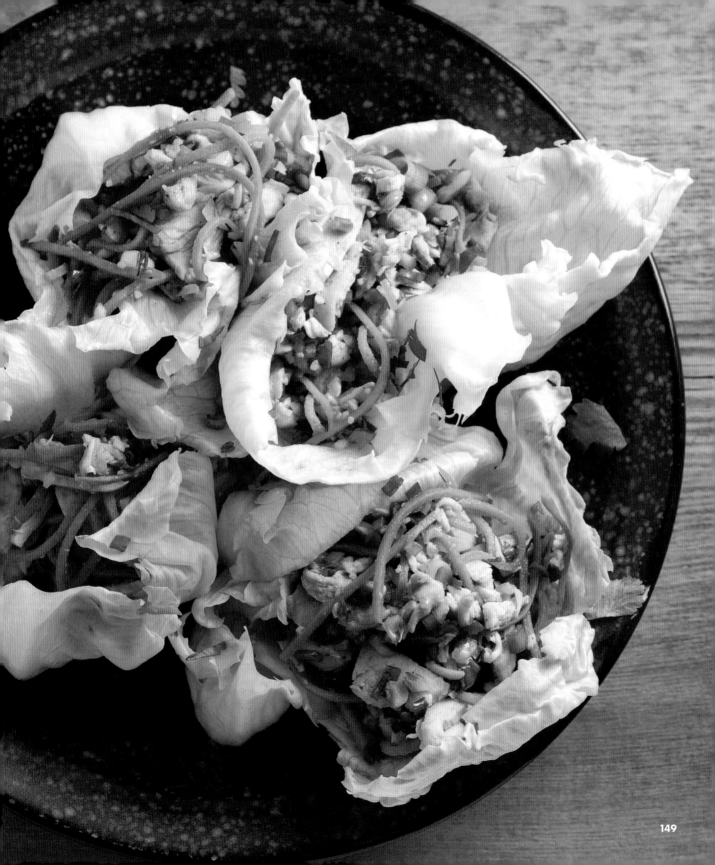

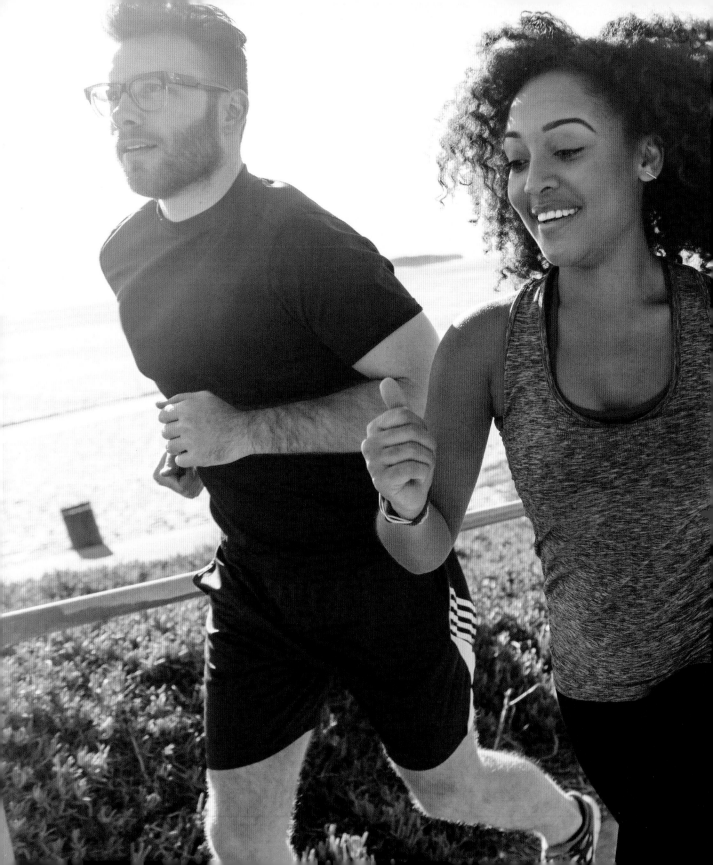

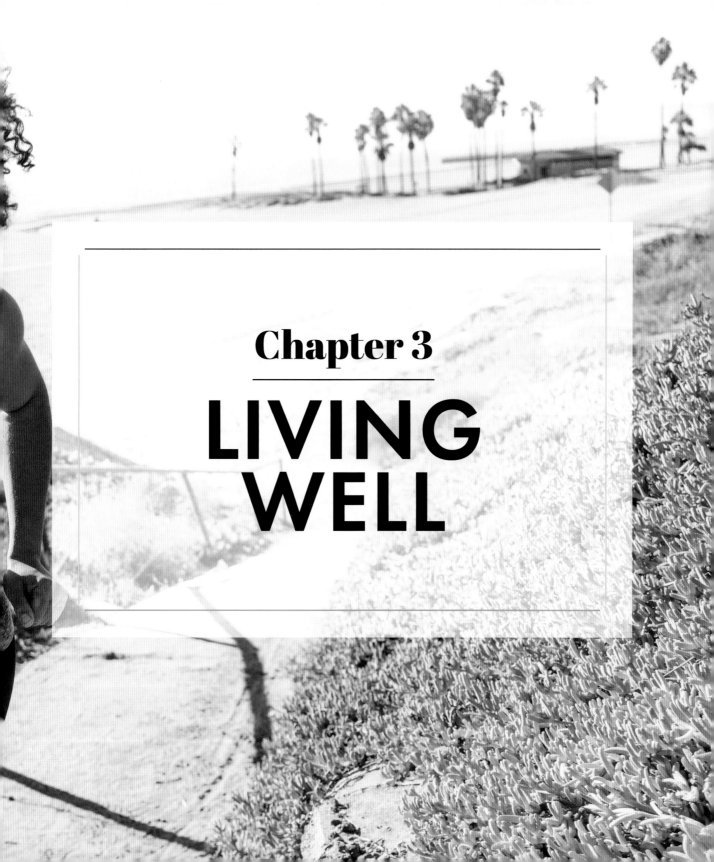

Chapter 3

LIVING WELL

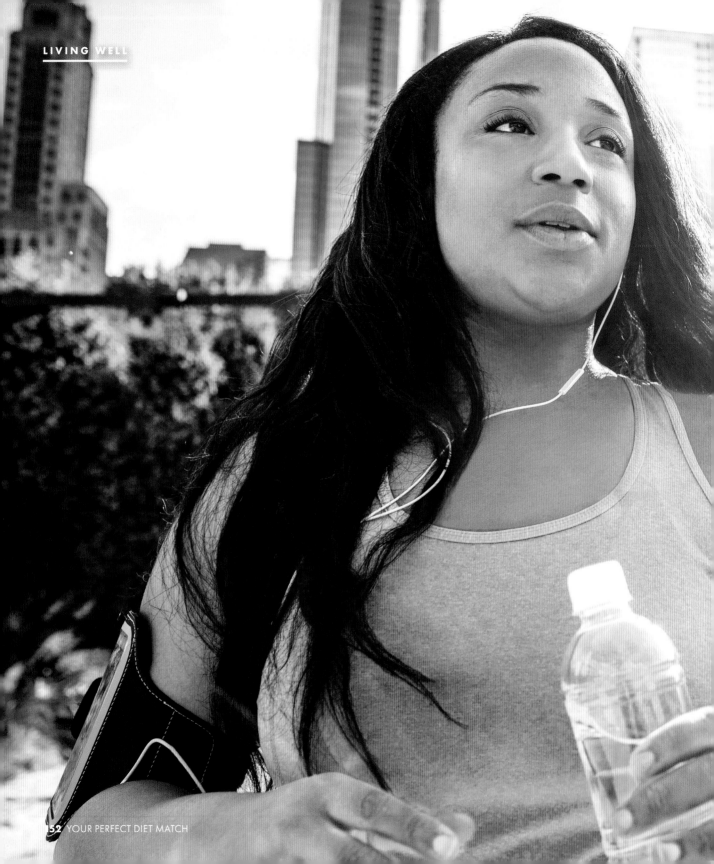

How Losing Weight Affects Your Health

Dropping even a few pounds can go a long way toward improving your well-being.

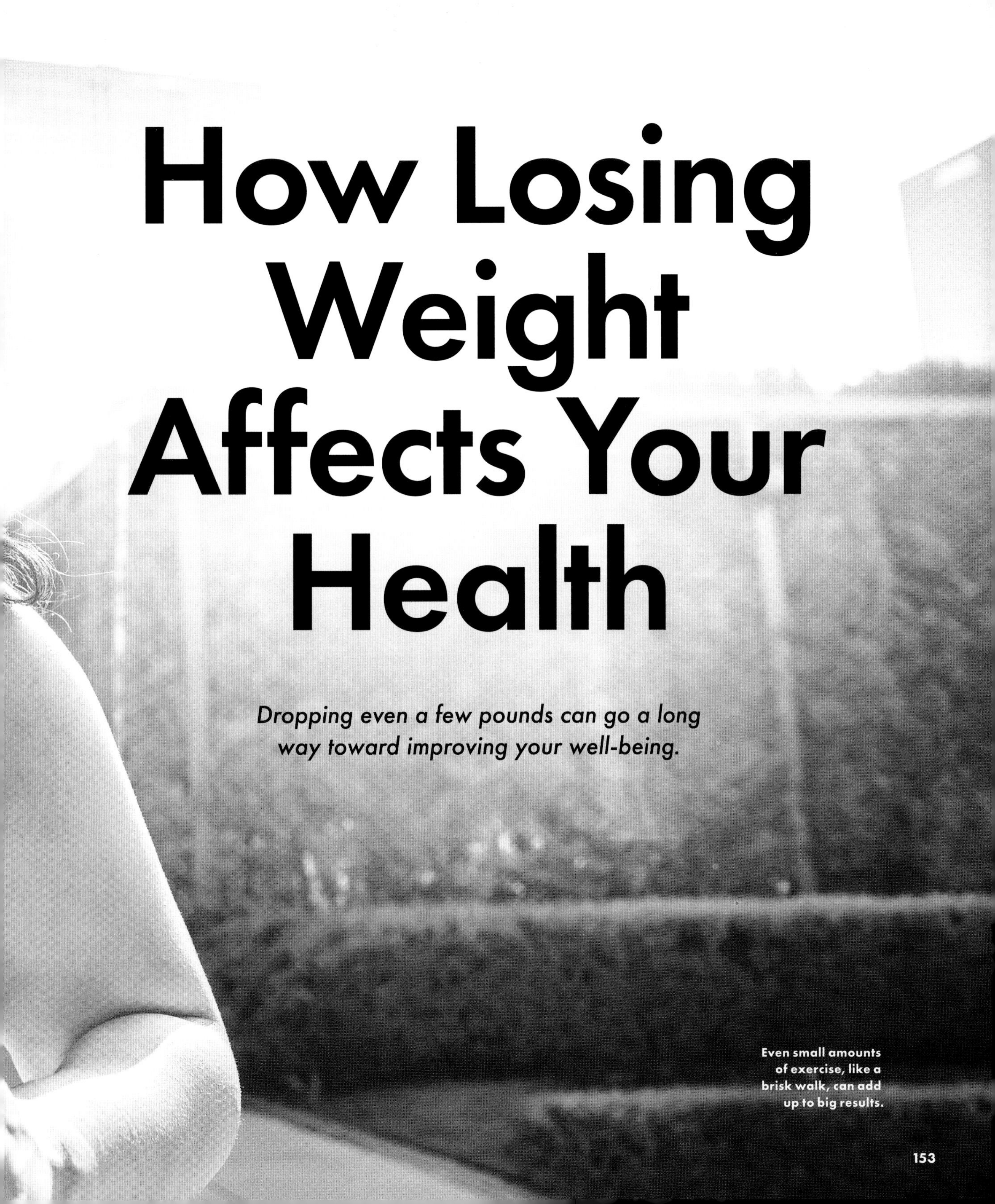

Even small amounts
of exercise, like a
brisk walk, can add
up to big results.

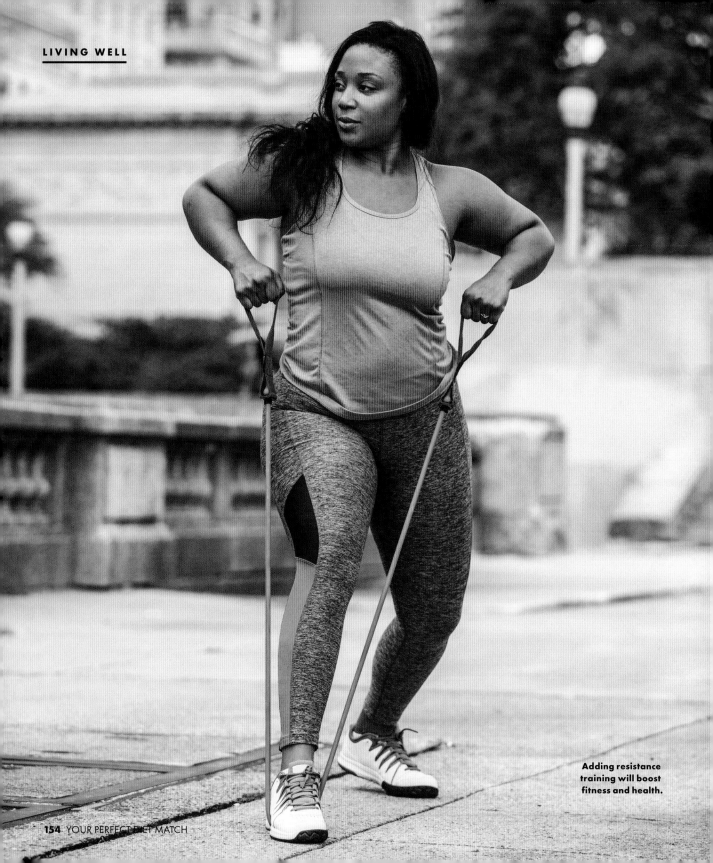

Adding resistance training will boost fitness and health.

N eed more motivation to lose weight than just looking better? Being overweight plays a role in two of our biggest killers—heart disease and cancer—as well as numerous other serious conditions. And obesity costs an estimated $350 billion annually in the U.S., according to a report in *Health Affairs*. But there's good news: Slimming down can have a major impact on your health—and we're not even talking *Biggest Loser*-esque pounds. Here, more reasons to drop some pounds.

Reduce Your Blood Pressure

Also known as hypertension, high blood pressure overworks the heart and contributes to arteriosclerosis (hardening of the arteries). It also increases the risk of heart disease and stroke, which are the first- and third-leading causes of death for Americans. High blood pressure is also linked to other serious conditions, such as congestive heart failure, kidney disease and blindness. The condition is closely correlated with how much you weigh—it rises as your body weight increases. The good news is that losing even 10 pounds can lower your blood pressure, a National Institutes of Health report found. The report went on to note that losing weight has the biggest effect on overweight people who already have hypertension.

Lower Your Cholesterol Levels

There are two sources of cholesterol: The first is your liver, which makes all the cholesterol your body needs (it's necessary for many vital bodily functions, such as building cells). The remainder of the cholesterol in your body comes from your diet, specifically animal products, like meat and dairy. Cholesterol can form a thick, waxy deposit on the inside of the arteries, which causes them to narrow and become less flexible (a condition known as atherosclerosis). If a blood clot forms and blocks one of these narrowed arteries, a heart attack or stroke can result, according to the American Heart Association. But even "a 5 percent weight loss improves cardiovascular risk factors," reducing your risk of having a heart attack or stroke, says Donna Arnett, Ph.D., dean of the University of Kentucky College of Public Health and a professor in the Department of Epidemiology and past president of the American Heart Association. And if you take medications to lower your cholesterol, losing weight may allow you to go off them (but consult with your doctor first).

Decrease Your Risk of Cancer

Being overweight is also strongly linked to an increased risk of cancer, according to research from the American Cancer Society. In fact, experts believe that about 7 percent of all cancer deaths in the U.S. are attributed to excess weight. It plays a role in breast, colon, esophageal, kidney and pancreatic cancers. Belly fat is linked with an increased risk of colon and rectal cancers.

Slash Your Chances of Getting Type 2 Diabetes

In a recent study published in *Cell Metabolism*, researchers discovered that as little as a 5 percent weight loss can improve metabolic disease, including insulin sensitivity and production, two of the leading risk factors for Type 2 diabetes. Also, losing weight can prevent diabetes' complications, such as blindness, kidney disease and limb amputation.

Say Goodbye to Back and Knee Pain

Excess weight puts extra stress on joints like knees and hips. Also, inflammation associated with weight gain is thought to contribute to trouble in other joints (for example, the hands). Losing a single pound results in 4 pounds of pressure being removed from the knees, a study in *Arthritis & Rheumatology* found. When you walk, the force on your knees is the equivalent of 1½ times your body weight, so losing 10 pounds would relieve 40 pounds of pressure from your knees.

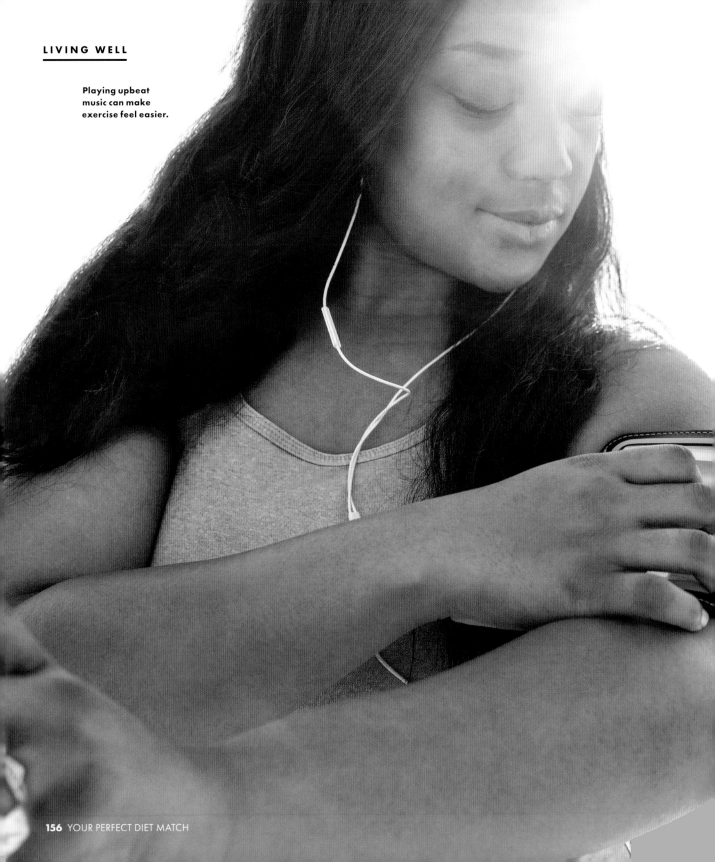

Playing upbeat music can make exercise feel easier.

A 200-pound man who lost 10 pounds would reduce the force on his knees by 22 percent, which could be enough to reverse painful knee issues.

And it's not just your lower body: Excess weight, especially around your middle, puts extra pressure on the vertebrae in your back, which can cause the vertebrae to become misaligned, resulting in back pain. In a 2012 study in *Arthritis & Rheumatology*, researchers found that disc degeneration tended to be more common and more severe among overweight or obese participants. Losing weight reduces pressure on the discs. Exercise plays a key role here: Not only can it can help you lose weight, but it will strengthen your back and abdominal muscles, which support your spine.

Sleep Better at Night

Do you snore, and do you find yourself nodding off during the day? You may have sleep apnea. With this condition, you stop breathing numerous times during the night, leading to poor-quality slumber and a constant feeling of being exhausted. Being overweight greatly increases the risk of sleep apnea, as fatty tissue around your airway obstructs your breathing. Also, when you're tired, you're more likely to overeat, and you're less likely to be motivated to exercise, creating a vicious cycle.

End Chronic Asthma Attacks

Even asthma symptoms can improve when you lose weight. When you are overweight or obese, most excess weight tends to settle around your midsection. This can reduce your lung volume, so you can't breathe as well, according to the American College of Allergy, Asthma & Immunology. Also, when you start eating a healthier diet, you're less likely to eat pro-inflammatory foods like sugary, starchy items. These can cause your body to release inflammatory hormones, such as leptin, that increase inflammation in the lungs and can lead to asthma attacks. By omitting them from your diet, you'll probably breathe easier.

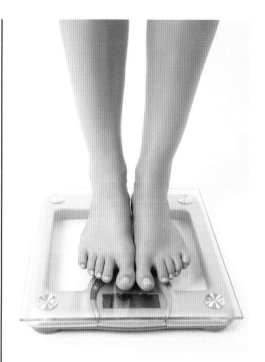

ALL IT TAKES IS 5 PERCENT

While losing 10 percent of your body weight is often touted as the threshold for seeing health benefits from weight loss, a 2016 Washington University study found that isn't necessarily the case. "Our findings demonstrate that you get the biggest bang for your buck with a 5 percent weight loss," said Samuel Klein, the director of the university's Center for Human Nutrition. "You don't have to lose 50 pounds to get important health benefits."

Although a few of the study's participants who went on to lose 10 percent of their body weight saw some increased benefits, those gains were minor compared to the changes they saw after losing 5 percent of their weight. "Losing 5 percent of your body weight is much easier than losing 10 percent," Klein says. "So it may make sense for patients to aim for [that] easier target."

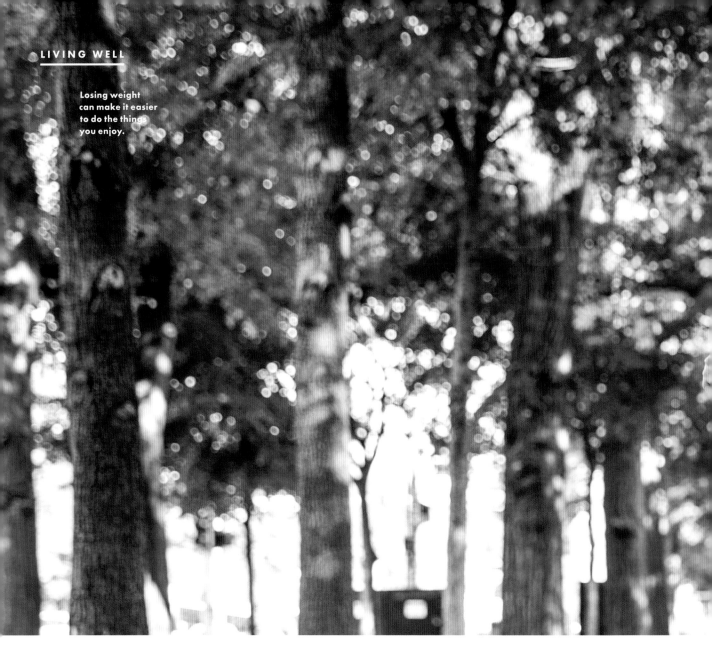

Losing weight can make it easier to do the things you enjoy.

Ditch the Heartburn Meds

The American Society for Gastrointestinal Endoscopy says that being overweight is a major cause of heartburn, also known as acid reflux and gastroesophageal reflux disease (GERD). It's caused when increased pressure in the abdomen causes stomach fluid to break through the barrier between the stomach and the esophagus. A 2014 study in *Obesity* found that 81 percent of participants in a six-month weight-loss program experienced a reduction in GERD symptoms, and 65 percent no longer had any reflux symptoms at all.

Prevent Cognitive Decline

Slimming down can have positive effects on brain health and may play a role in the prevention of

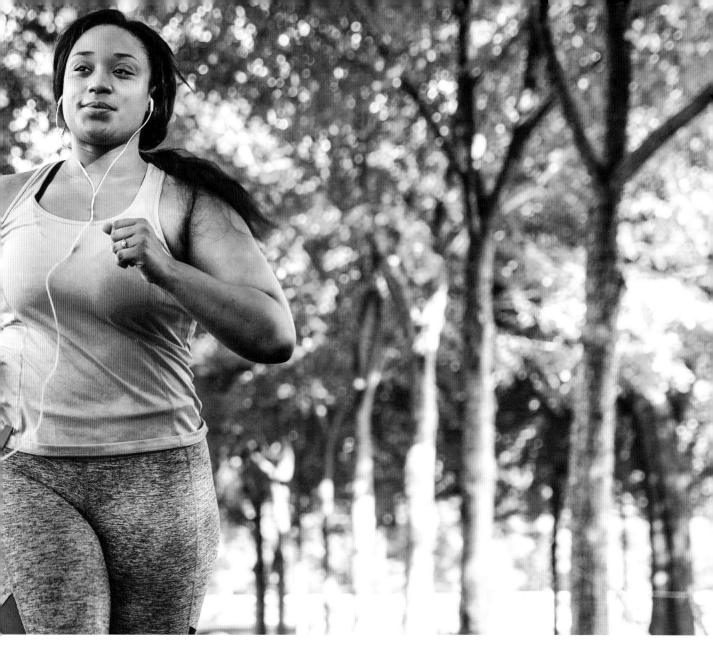

cognitive degeneration and age-related dementia, including Alzheimer's disease. A 2012 study in *Neurology* found that brain function was lower in people who have too many extra pounds. And researchers at Brazil's University of São Paulo found that obese participants who lost weight did as well on cognitive tests as lean women in the control group.

Put an End to Exhaustion

When you're lugging around fewer pounds, you have more energy and stamina to get through your day, whether it's going for a run in the morning or doing housework at night. After all, more body weight can translate into more work, even when it comes to things like climbing stairs. Lighten that load and you'll feel less fatigued!

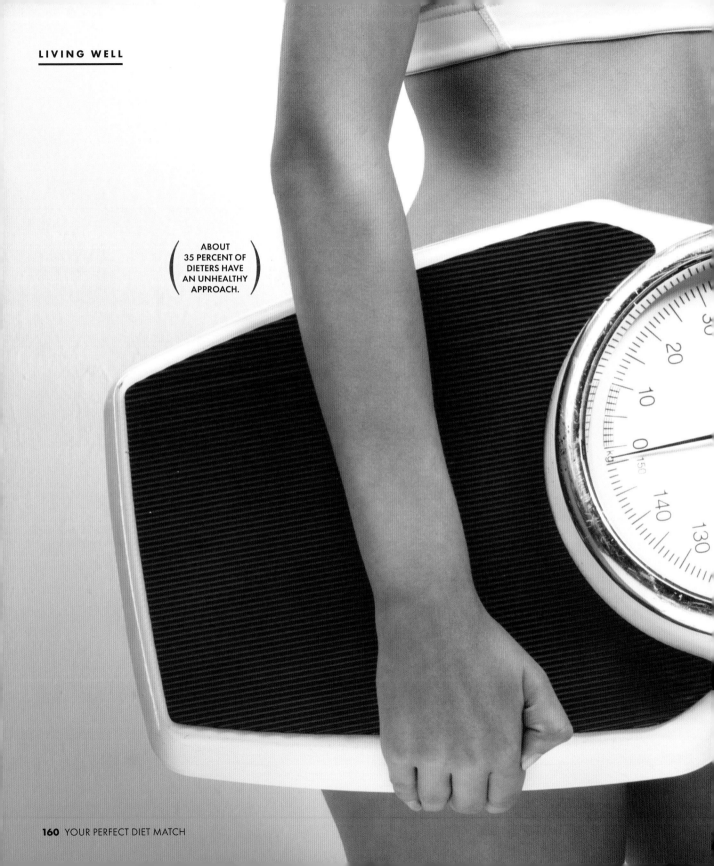

ABOUT
35 PERCENT OF
DIETERS HAVE
AN UNHEALTHY
APPROACH.

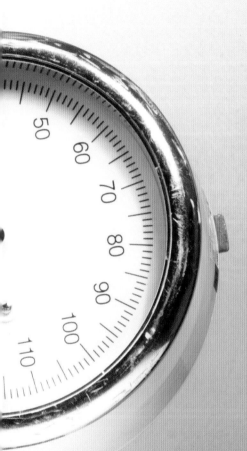

When Dieting Goes Too Far

How to know when your weight-loss attempts have gotten the better of you—and what to do if you've lost control.

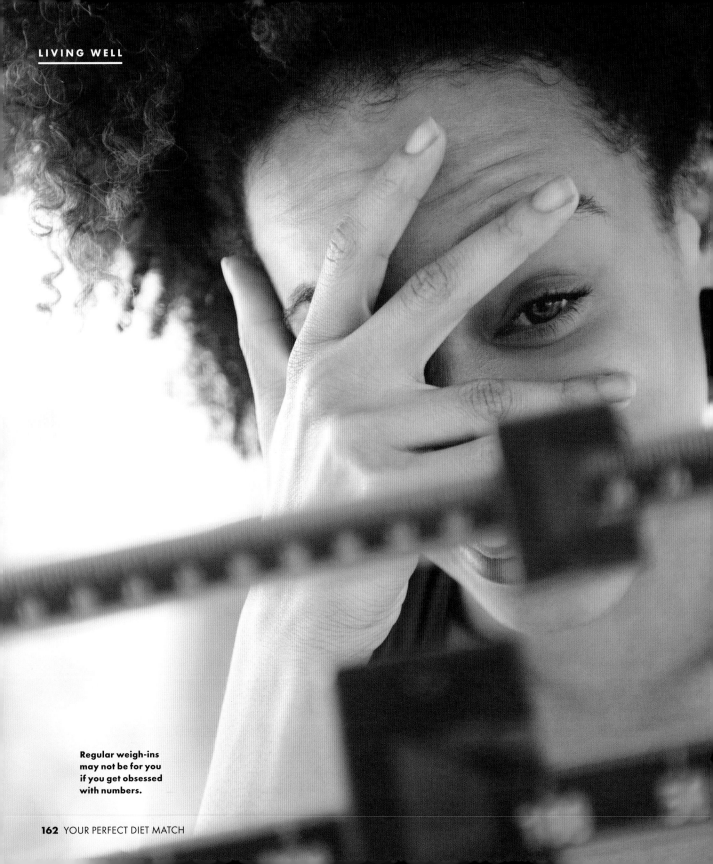

Regular weigh-ins
may not be for you
if you get obsessed
with numbers.

At 12 years old I didn't know what role carbs played in keeping my body healthy. I just assumed they were bad. I'd watched my mother diet for most of my childhood, and while she never suggested I follow her lead, her eschewing of bread, restriction of calories, and the tension she expressed at the dining table were easy to model. Since elementary school, I'd felt debilitating self-consciousness about the size of my stomach and the shape of my face. I feared myself to be too large to be lovable. It dawned on me that by not eating I could control my appearance. In high school, I started restricting my food intake and exercising off as many calories as I could. This continued into my 20s. I'd stopped menstruating and all my energy was directed at calculating how and when I'd eat or exercise next. To the outside world, I was a paragon of health, sticking to a laudable diet and exercise regimen. It wasn't until I sought treatment for an eating disorder in college that I developed a healthier relationship with nutrition and physical activity. But after so many years spent alienating myself from my body's real needs, it's taken me almost a decade to re-learn how to nourish myself in a truly healthy way.

Unfortunately, I'm not alone. According to the National Eating Disorders Association, an estimated 20 million American women and 10 million American men will develop an eating disorder during their lifetime. Here's how to tell if your eating regimen's gotten the better of you—and how to get help if it has.

Does a Healthy Diet Exist?

"Most popular diets geared toward weight loss, especially rapid weight loss, are inherently a little disordered," says New York City–based therapist Catherine Silver, L.C.S.W., who specializes in treating eating disorders and body-image issues. "Typically they don't encourage you to listen to your body, which is really the only healthy way to lose weight."

Because diets often teach us to follow a calculated plan rather than tune into our body's needs, they can alienate us from our body's own natural hunger and fullness signals and start a dangerous cycle of yo-yo dieting that puts our physical and emotional well-being at risk, Silver explains. What's worse, she adds, is that our culture has largely normalized a slew of unhealthy approaches to eating that many diet trends entail—so much so that many of us consider some seriously disordered behaviors. For example, we eliminate entire food groups such as grains or dairy when we don't have a food allergy.

Or consider the connotations that trendy diets graft onto different categories of food—"good" versus "bad" carbohydrates, for instance, which implies that you're doing something naughty if you dare indulge in the latter; or the concept of "clean" eating, which casts a range of edibles that might not be so bad for you if consumed in moderation as "dirty." All of this, Silver notes, can make the basic human experience of nourishing our bodies seem like a battleground of good and evil.

We can even overdo it on supposedly "healthy eating." Orthorexia is a fancy term for an obsessive and all-consuming preoccupation with this way of eating that interferes with a person's emotional, social, sometimes professional, and often physical well-being. (Refusing to eat anything that's not organic, for instance, can get in the way of enjoying your life, and put you at risk for nutrient deficiencies.)

This doesn't mean that preferring to buy wild-caught salmon at the market or making sure that you keep candy bars out of your snack drawer means you've got a problem. But if you're stuck for an extended amount of time in a place where the only edible options fall outside your dietary regimen's rules and you opt to go hungry while anxiety grips you in a cold sweat? That's where the difference between passion and pathology lies, says Silver.

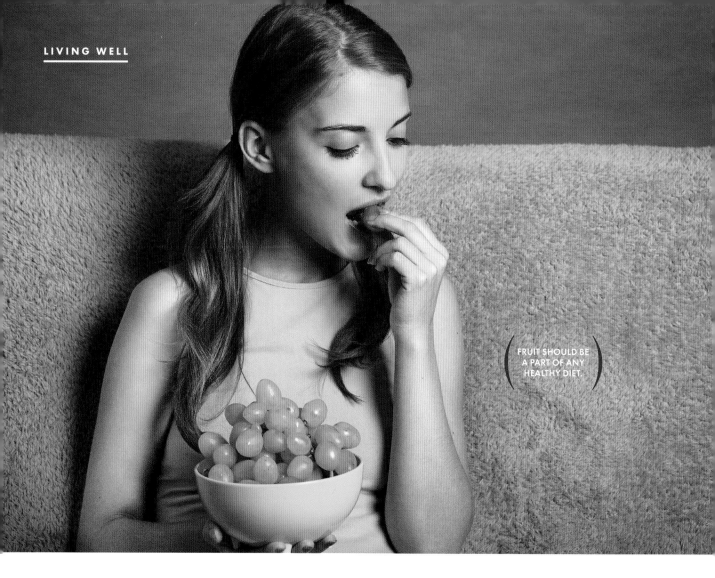

FRUIT SHOULD BE
A PART OF ANY
HEALTHY DIET.

If You Have Crossed a Line

It took me herniating two discs in my back and stress fractures in both my feet from overexercising and depriving my body of key nutrients to finally ask myself: What was I doing this for—and how much longer could I survive if I kept it up? As my preoccupation with staying thin encroached on just about every aspect of my life (work, friendships, my dating life) I knew I had to get help or risk being miserable for the rest of my life.

Whether your diet is healthy or harmful boils down to the physical and emotional consequences it comes with, says Silver. If you're wondering whether yours is veering into unhealthy territory, consider asking the following: How much is your diet getting in the way of the rest of your life? What happens when you deviate from your diet? Do you beat yourself up? If the food rules you're following are precluding you from enjoying activities you once loved or spending time with people who mean something to you, or are dominating your every decision as well as how great or horrible you feel in your skin, you may need to start rethinking your relationship with food.

Pay attention as well to the physical signs that your diet is doing your body more harm than good, adds Silver. Fractures, extreme fatigue, dizziness (especially when standing after sitting), irritability, digestive issues (constipation, bloating or diarrhea)—and, in more extreme cases, heart palpitations and chest pains that crop up after you've radically altered your eating habits—are serious signs what you're doing is not good for your long-term health.

So…What Actually Works?

What might a healthy eating plan look like, by comparison? "A sound approach to nutrition is flexible, not guided by extreme rules or guidelines, is heavy on the veggies, lean proteins, complex carbs (like beans and whole grains), and healthy fats (avocados, olive oil), but not to the total exclusion of other foods," says Bari Stricoff, R.D.N, L.D.N., who specializes in eating-disorder nutrition therapy. No, dessert at every meal might not help you fit into those skinny jeans, but consuming it in moderation isn't going to wreck your waistline—or your health. Being able to nosh on delectable goodies sans guilt and without losing control is a major hallmark of a healthy approach to nutrition, Stricoff says.

How to Get Help

There's no shame in reaching out for help. Here are some organizations:
• National Eating Disorders Association (NEDA). Call 1-800-931-2237 or visit their website at: nationaleatingdisorders.org
• Binge Eating Disorder Association (BEDA). Visit their website at: eatingdisorderhope.com
• National Association of Anorexia Nervosa and Associated Disorders (ANAD). Call their helpline at 630-577-1330 or visit: anad.org
• International Association of Eating Disorder Professionals (IAEDP). Visit their website at: iaedp.com
• Project HEAL is a fundraising organization that can help fund treatment for an eating disorder. Visit: theprojectheal.org

—*Katherine Schreiber*

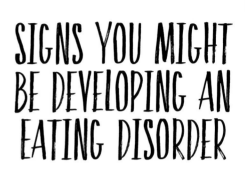

SIGNS YOU MIGHT BE DEVELOPING AN EATING DISORDER

Eating disorders come in many different forms. Signs you may be struggling with one include excessive preoccupation with weight, shape or size, or the "health" or "cleanliness" of food, and extreme or rigid rituals and rules about food, says Neeru Bakshi, M.D., medical director at Eating Recovery Center Washington (located in Bellevue and Seattle).

The Diagnostic and Statistical Manual of Mental Disorders-5 (the tome mental health professionals rely on to categorize psychiatric conditions) currently recognizes eight categories of eating disorders, Bakshi says. Here are three of the most common ones:

• **Anorexia** Involves the restriction of energy intake coupled with a fear of gaining weight and "a disturbance in the way someone experiences their weight or body shape," Bakshi explains.

• **Binge-Eating Disorder** Repeated episodes of extreme overeating resulting in high levels of emotional distress.

• **Bulimia** Symptoms include "recurrent binge-eating and inappropriate compensatory behaviors to try and prevent weight gain," Bakshi says. These can include self-induced vomiting, taking laxatives or forcing yourself to run because you ate dessert.

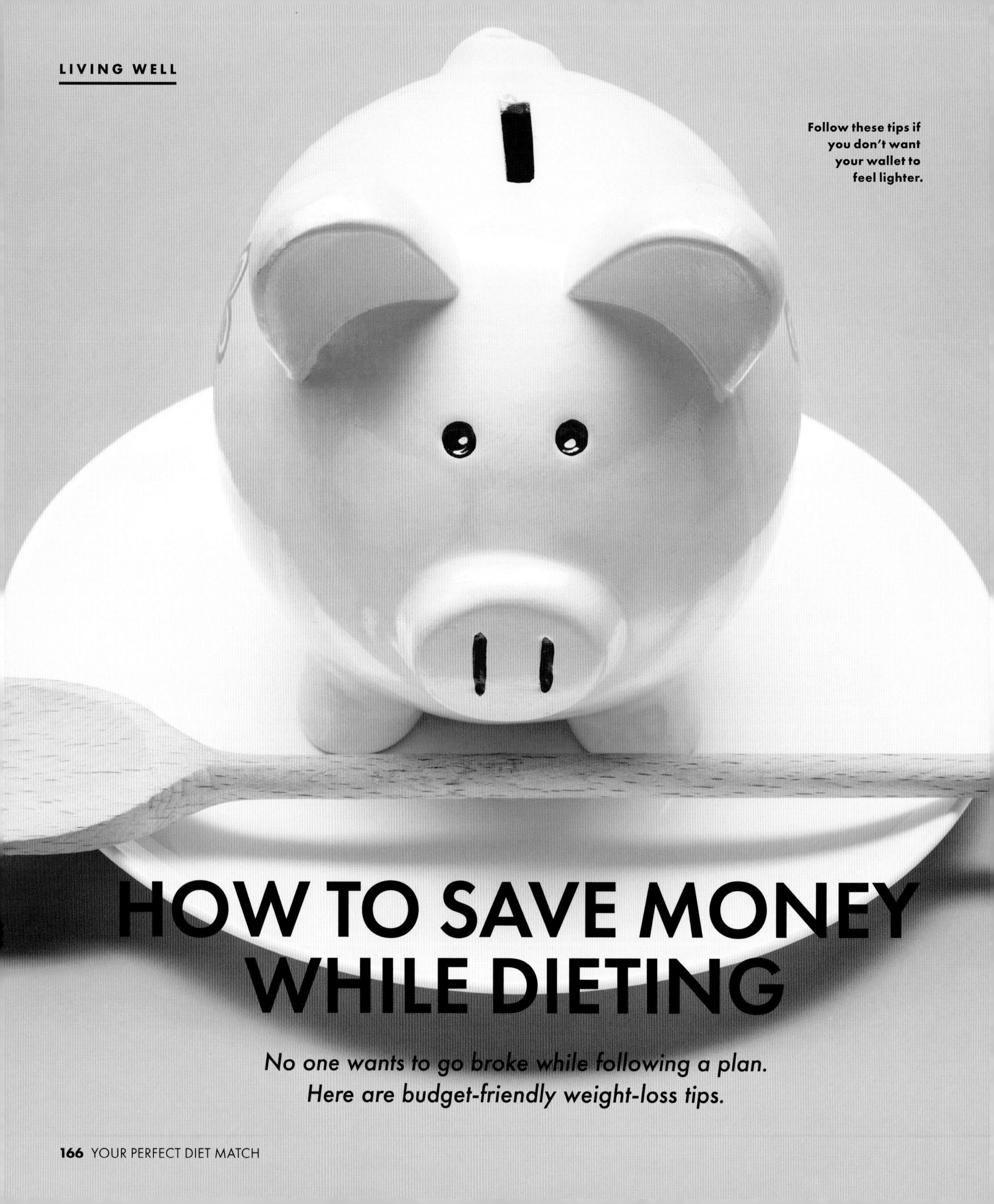

Follow these tips if
you don't want
your wallet to
feel lighter.

HOW TO SAVE MONEY
WHILE DIETING

No one wants to go broke while following a plan.
Here are budget-friendly weight-loss tips.

Some diets can be followed by researching the plan online (like keto, Paleo, DASH and the Mediterranean diet, for example); others have a lot of rules and will be easier if you buy a book, like *The Dubrow Diet* or *The Lose Your Belly Diet*. And some have an ongoing membership program you'll pay for, like Noom or WW.

And while you'll have to buy different foods, healthy eating doesn't have to cost a lot of money if you know what to buy and how to find deals. "When you pay attention to what you are eating, you begin to eat less and can save money while losing," says weight-loss expert Liz Josefsberg, C.P.T., author of *Target 100*.

Here are a few different money-saving ideas to help you stick to a budget as you shed pounds.

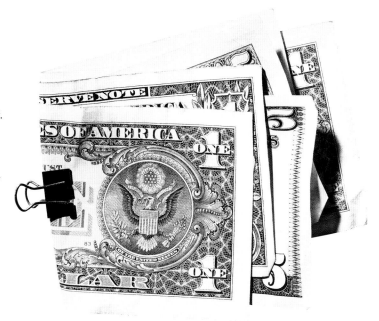

How to Save on Any Diet

GO HALFSIES When dining out, cut portions in half and have the leftovers for lunch the next day. You'll essentially cut your price (and calories consumed) in half.

CURB ALCOHOL "In order to lose weight, you will need to seriously consider your alcohol intake," says Josefsberg. Cutting way back will save money and amp up weight loss.

PLAN AND PREP MEALS Create a menu for the week so you can shop according to that list and portion out foods so you don't overeat, or overbuy.

BROWN BAG IT Bringing lunch from home will save money and calories. It'll be easier to stick to your diet instead of wandering the minefield of restaurants near your workplace.

PRACTICE BYOB Fill a water bottle at home and keep it with you when you're on the go to stay hydrated and save money instead of purchasing bottled H2O.

How to Save on a Plant-Based Diet

SHOP THE FREEZER AISLE Flash-frozen fruits and veggies are as nutritious as fresh, says Vanessa Voltolina, M.S., R.D.N.

STOCK UP ON SELECT SEASONAL PRODUCE Buy the best-priced items based upon the season and their availability.

BUY SHELF STABLE ITEMS DURING SALES Beans are a good option for a healthy canned food that provides protein and fiber. Drain and rinse canned beans first to reduce sodium.

How to Save on a Low-Carb Diet

THINK BIG Purchase meat in family packs at a wholesale club. "Making one smart, lean protein in a way that can be used all week will save you money," suggests Josefsberg.

INVEST IN A SPIRALIZER Make "zoodles" from zucchini and "coodles" from carrots at home so you're not spending extra on those precut packaged versions.

GO NUTS! Buy almonds or other nuts in bulk (available on Amazon or clubs like Costco). Use a food processor to make your own nut butters and you can save approximately 50 percent over the store-bought versions.

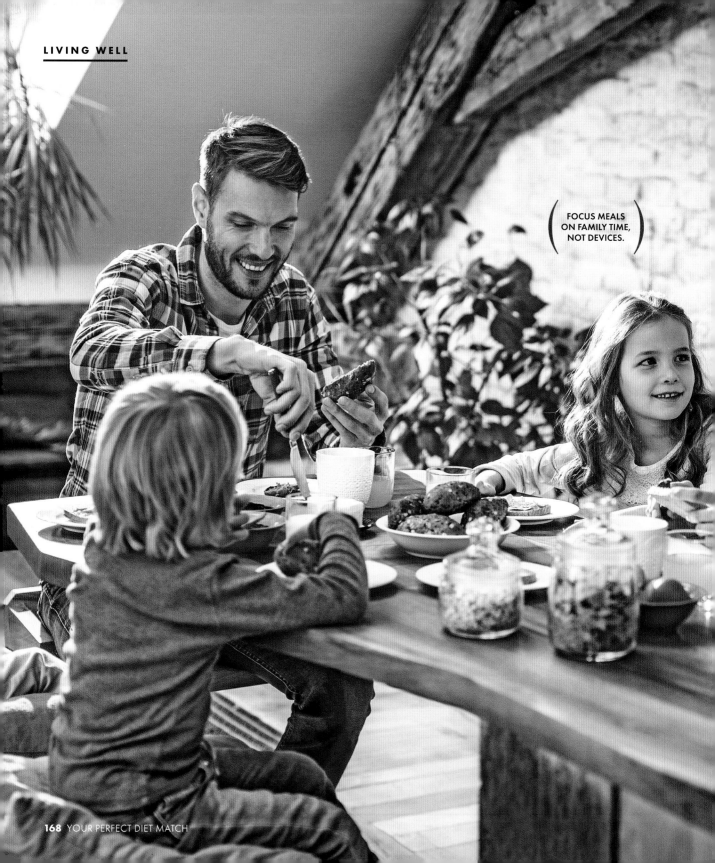

FOCUS MEALS ON FAMILY TIME, NOT DEVICES.

The Art of Eating Mindfully

Enjoy your food more and reap the benefits of a healthier diet (and smaller waistline!) by slowing down and savoring each bite.

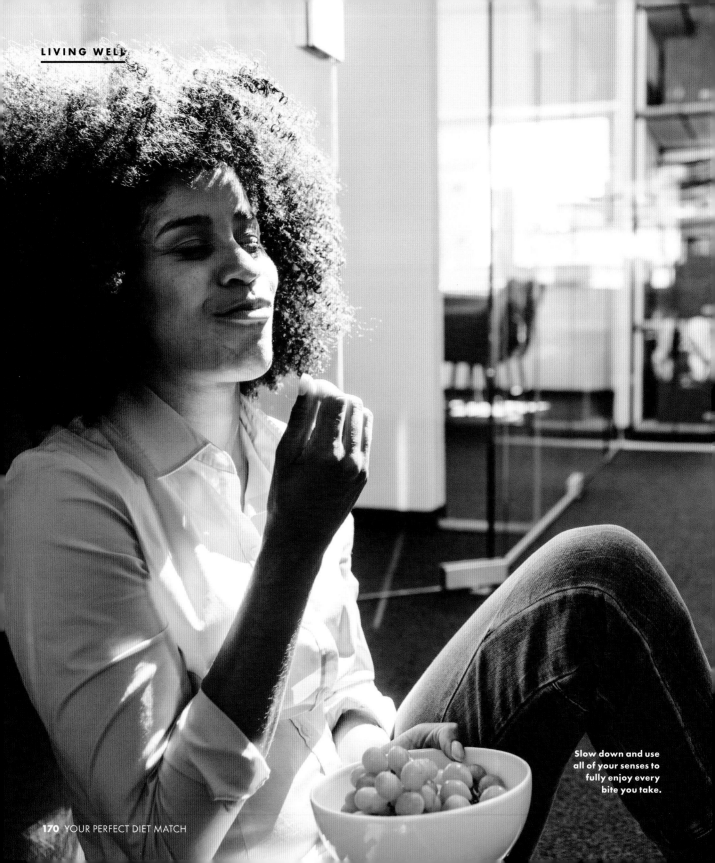

Slow down and use
all of your senses to
fully enjoy every
bite you take.

Whether you're constantly looking for the next great diet or just want to focus on the foods that will help you stay healthy, minding what you eat is important. But are you really being mindful about what you eat?

All too often, many of us will sit in front of a screen or in a car and mindlessly munch away. Whether you're chewing a sandwich or shoveling down a bowl of spaghetti, you're probably not paying attention to what you're putting in your mouth. And that can lead to overeating and, eventually, weight gain, along with other health concerns. With one out of every three individuals in America classified as obese, it's likely that much of the problem can be linked to our bad habit of distracted eating, says Joyce Faraj, Ph.D., R.D.N., a nutritionist at Mountainside Treatment Center in Canaan, Connecticut. "A lot of us are guilty of eating while we're at our desks or watching TV, or simply eating as a means to an end and not really paying attention to what we're putting in our bodies or how much we're consuming," she notes. As a result, she says, the average daily intake of calories for an American is more than 3,000— "which is a lot more than most of us need."

After all, it's fairly easy to down a whole bag of chips while binge-watching Netflix, or polish off a carton of ice cream as you finish up a project in front of the computer. That's because your brain doesn't fully register what you're eating, so you don't get the same satiety cues, explains Karen Koenig, M.Ed., a specialist in eating psychology in Sarasota, Florida, and the author of *Helping Patients Outsmart Overeating*. It takes about 20 minutes for the brain to register hormonal signals from the gut that it's full; eat too quickly, and those cues can become garbled.

"When we don't put attention on what we are eating, our bodies don't register satisfaction, which is quality-based, and fullness, which is quantity-based. This makes us more likely to eat more food, more frequently," Koenig explains.

"We don't chew slowly enough to release flavor, and we don't allow time for food to sit on our tongues so that our taste buds can send information to our brains to let it know whether we're full or satisfied."

Enter mindful eating—essentially, eating with awareness. At its core, mindful eating means engaging all of your senses as you eat: noting how your food looks and smells, its texture, and of course its taste. Then there's the process of eating itself: chewing slowly, without distractions like electronics or even reading.

The payoff? You'll enjoy your meals more, and your waistline will benefit both in the short- and long-term. In fact, a recent review by the National Institutes of Health showed that mindful eating played a strong role in both successfully losing weight and also in keeping it off, with a direct relationship between mindful eating and the reduction of food cravings, portion control, body mass index and body weight.

Ready to give it a try? For your next meal, try following these six simple rules for mindful eating.

1 Put Away Your Devices

Mindful eating is about focusing on just one thing at a time, so shelve your to-do list, step away from the computer, put down your phone and close your book. Find a pleasant place to eat, whether that's a park bench at lunchtime or a seat in your kitchen, and let your mind start to focus on the process of eating.

2 Go Slow

Set a timer for 20 minutes, then take all of that time to eat a normal-size meal. Slowing down makes you more mindful of what you're doing and really makes you focus on what you are eating, says Faraj. It might help to hold the fork in your nondominant hand or to try using chopsticks to emphasize this less-hurried pace. You can also try putting your fork down after each bite or taking frequent sips of water to cleanse your palate.

FIND YOUR PERFECT PORTION

"Portion control is a huge part of mindful eating," says health and wellness coach Rachel Gersten. Measuring out your food and sticking to that allotted portion not only helps your waistline, it will also allow you to better appreciate each bite you take. Follow this guide to keep your portions in perspective.

SERVING SIZE EQUALS

1 cup cereal	Your fist
1 pancake	Compact disc
½ cup cooked rice	Half of a baseball
3 ounces meat	Deck of cards
3 ounces fish	Checkbook
Salad	Two fists
Slice of bread	Flat hand
1 spoon of peanut butter	Thumb

3 Savor Each Bite

Take a few seconds to examine your food, smell it and savor that first bite as you start chewing. Are you eating something crunchy, like celery? How does that feel in your mouth, against your teeth? Or are you eating something smooth, like yogurt? Notice the way it feels against your tongue. Continue to take small bites, chewing well and enjoying the different textures and flavor.

4 Tune in to Your Body

"Halfway through your meal, ask yourself if you are still hungry or whether you are reaching a point of satisfaction where you could stop eating and be OK," says Faraj. "Really listen to your body, and stop eating when you feel neutral—not stuffed."

Then think about how you feel when your meal is done. Do you feel bloated or tired after having a plate of fries or half the bread basket? Does a salad full of fresh vegetables help you feel energized? Listening to your body's cues after eating specific foods is a key component of mindful eating, she adds.

5 Plan Out Your Meals

Know roughly what you are going to eat for the next few days by planning out all of your main meals. "Write down what you want to make for breakfast, lunch and dinner for the entire week," suggests Rachel Gersten, a New York City therapist and health/wellness coach. "This way, you'll make sure you're eating a balanced diet and getting in the right mix of nutrients."

6 Avoid Emotional Eating

Stress eating can counter all of the mindful gains you've made thus far, so it's important to find other ways to combat the stress in your life during the day, Koenig says. Plan regular workouts, talk on the phone with your friend, do a crossword, head out for a walk. "Find effective skills to cope with life's ups and downs without turning to food," she says.

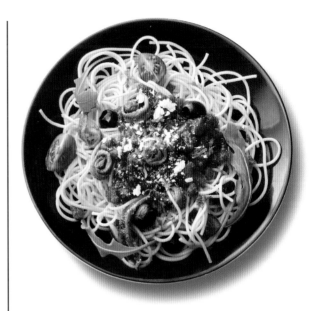

EATING BY THE NUMBERS

20 minutes
Amount of time it takes for the message to get to your brain that your stomach is full

1 out of 3
Portion of Americans defined as obese

3,600
Average number of calories an American eats in a given day

1,600–2,600
Average amount of calories recommended per day, based on gender and activity level

The Importance of Exercise

Physical activity is paramount for keeping weight off and stoking your metabolism. Here's why.

The mood-boosting benefits of exercise will carry through your day.

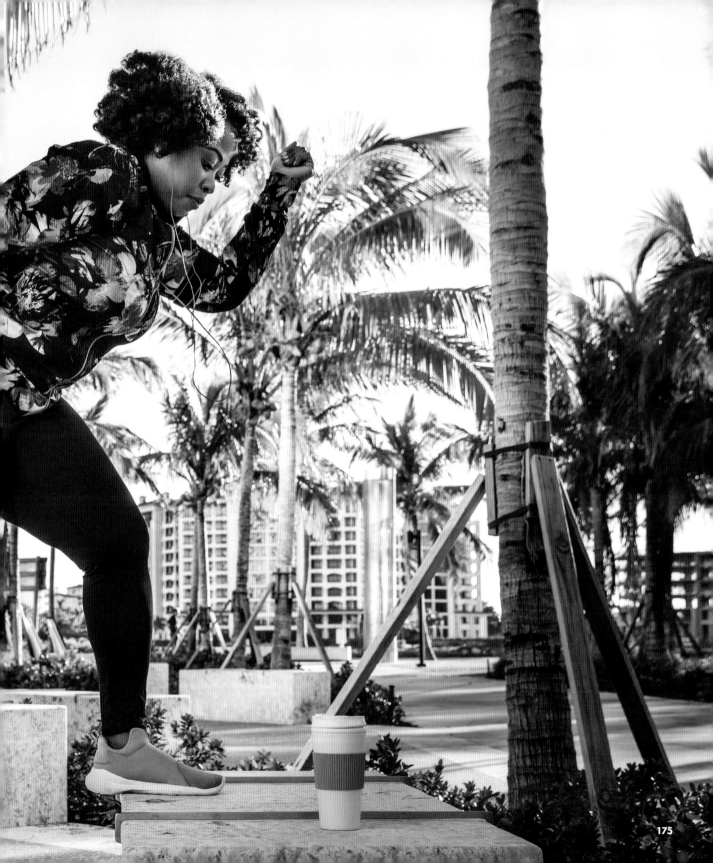

Y ou know by now that a diet that consists of you and a few carrot sticks isn't going to get you too far in terms of lasting success: It takes balanced meal plans with reasonable calorie restrictions to drop excess pounds and keep them off. But what role does exercise play when it comes to weight loss? Turns out, quite a bit—especially if you want your results to stick. Exercise has a number of crucial benefits, from burning calories and preserving lean muscle to curbing appetite and improving self-esteem. But all exercise isn't created equal when it comes to weight loss. What you do, how much of it and in what combination all matter. Here, we explore some of the more common myths about how weight loss and exercise work together, and how to find the balance that will suit you best.

MYTH 1 Weight Loss Is Only About Calories in Versus Calories Out

Eating more calories than you're burning off? It's true, you're not going to lose weight— regardless of how intense your workout regimen is. But what you are eating is just as important as how much you consume.

"The biggest [component of weight loss] is what you put into your body," says Liz Lowe, C.S.C.S. "If you're constantly eating empty calories from processed foods with added sugars and fats, you won't have the proper fuel to power your workouts."

And it's not as black-and-white as "calories in versus calories out" either. "People are disconnected from what and how much they eat and the difference between hunger and fullness," says Mary Jane Detroyer, R.D.N., P.T., who specializes in weight-loss management. Step away from the scale and shift your mindset from being only motivated by pounds lost. "In the beginning, focus on your behaviors and your ability to be consistent—that's how you get results," she notes.

Likewise, resist the impulse to go for the fast fix. Most transformations take months or even

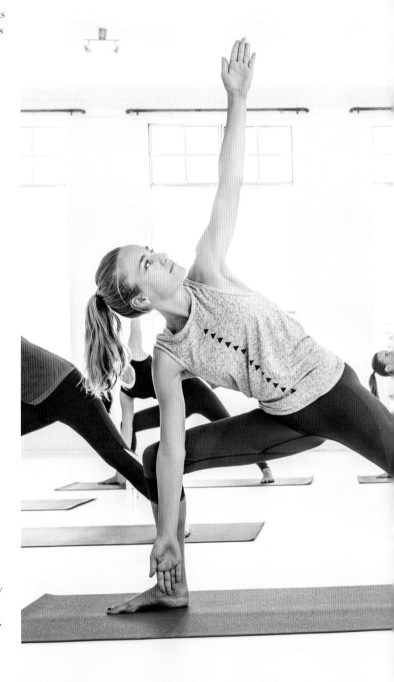

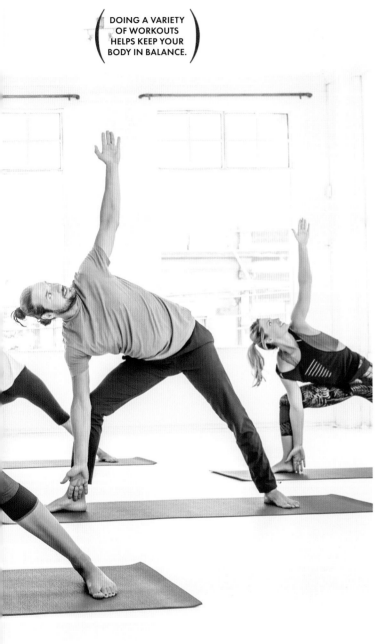

years of sustained effort. For safe, sustainable weight loss, stick to the rule of 1 to 2 pounds a week, Lowe says: "That's a deficit of 3,500 to 7,000 calories per week. If you go much under that, you're going to slow down your metabolism." Too much deprivation will stress out your body and trigger it to enter starvation mode, a fail-safe measure that makes it harder to lose weight and can turn your body catabolic, so it starts to break down lean muscle tissue.

"One of the best ways to get into a caloric deficit without consuming an abnormally low amount of food is through proper exercise—especially intense exercise, which includes strength training and high-intensity and steady-state cardio, as well as plenty of daily activity mixed in," says Joel Seedman, Ph.D. "Walking is one of the most underrated ways to ditch unwanted fat, prolong longevity and improve fitness."

MYTH 2 Cardio Alone Is the Best Way to Drop Extra Pounds

Many of us decide to adopt cardio workouts when we're starting a weight-loss program. While some think running is the best go-to for dropping pounds, if you're overweight or obese, your doctor probably recommends low-impact, low-intensity cardio, like walking or cycling on a stationary bike.

But eventually, that all-cardio routine will cause you to hit a plateau, Seedman says. That's because you'll be losing both fat and muscle. "You've got to challenge the cardiovascular and musculoskeletal systems," he adds. "Until you have enough lean muscle mass on your body, it's going to be tough to reach your optimal weight and body composition." Doing resistance exercise is important for weight loss, since it helps preserve muscle mass.

Muscle is naturally metabolic, meaning it burns more calories both when it's being used and at rest, Detroyer explains. "People who have more muscle tend to burn more calories during workouts and can push themselves harder."

There's no set formula that computes how much more muscle you need to burn a specific number of calories, but every little bit helps.

Strength and resistance training can also help ramp up your metabolism as it slows, which may be much earlier than you think. "Research indicates that everyone's metabolism starts dropping somewhere around their early to mid- or late 20s," Seedman says.

MYTH 3 Exercise Alone Is Enough to Help You Lose Weight

The majority of randomized, controlled trials indicate that people experience only moderate weight loss with either exercise or diet alone, according to materials published in *Nature Reviews Endocrinology*. Combining activity with dietary changes substantially boosts the odds of successful long-term weight loss. And experts maintain this combo is essential for overweight and obese individuals to maintain their losses. A big hurdle with exercise is sticking to it; most people don't, because it feels like a chore or a punishment. If you struggle with motivation and accountability, look for a community-based weight-loss program for support.

MYTH 4 Exercise Will Make You Tired

Yes, we've all heard this excuse as a reason people don't want to work out. But paradoxically, when you exercise your body releases endorphins, which help boost your mood and make you feel energized. Harder workouts, like HIIT (high-intensity interval training), may produce a stronger endorphin release, according to research from the University of Turku in Finland. And if you feel lethargic or sluggish, exercise can help by improving insulin function. "Because of the American diet and sedentary lifestyle, most people don't absorb carbs, or nutrients in general, all that well," Seedman says. A lot of the nutrients in food end up hanging out in the bloodstream or get shuttled to fat cells. But when you train, your muscles compete for those nutrients. "More efficient fat and sugar metabolism mean a reduced risk of heart disease and diabetes," Detroyer adds.

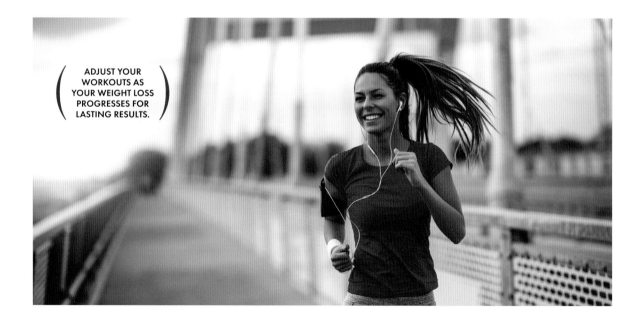

ADJUST YOUR WORKOUTS AS YOUR WEIGHT LOSS PROGRESSES FOR LASTING RESULTS.

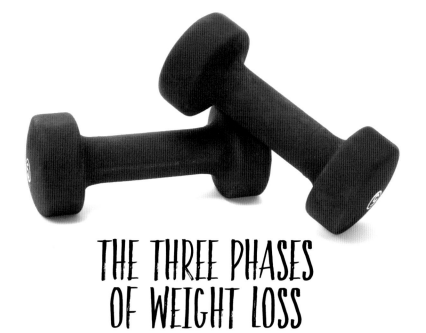

THE THREE PHASES OF WEIGHT LOSS

Phase I
Initial Weight Loss

"If you've never exercised before, increase your activity levels to two to three times per week," says trainer Liz Lowe, C.S.C.S. Go for a walk. Do laps in a pool. Work with a personal trainer and learn the basics of strength training. "After a couple of weeks, ramp it up to three times a week, then four, and slowly build your duration and intensity," she says. You don't want to burn yourself out or get injured.

Phase II
Continued Weight Loss, Body-Composition Changes

"Strength training prevents the body from breaking down muscle and helps promote fat loss at the same time—especially in people who do a lot of cardio," says Joel Seedman, Ph.D. And your body needs that muscle for weight-loss success. "One extra pound of muscle on your body can help you burn anywhere from five to 50 calories per day," Seedman says. "Exercise helps prevent muscle loss that can occur as you lose weight, builds lean mass, ensures the metabolism doesn't slow down, and preserves endocrine function by regulating hormones." Specifically, exercise boosts testosterone, lowers cortisol and improves insulin function. But just pumping iron isn't the best option, either: "People who only strength train tend to hold a little too much body fat, so a combination of one or two high-intensity workouts a week can speed up a sluggish metabolism," Seedman explains. It's recommended that healthy individuals aim for 150 minutes of moderate-intensity cardio exercise weekly. Break that up into five 30-minute sessions, or log longer weekend workouts.

Phase III
Maintenance

To keep the weight off, you have to increase your resting metabolic rate, which is the number of calories your body burns at rest. The only way to do that is to build lean muscle, Lowe says.

Exercise is the single strongest predictor of weight-loss maintenance, according to a meta-analysis published in *Obesity*, which reviewed studies including men, women, adolescents and massively obese populations. Those who underwent supervised 40-minute training sessions—hitting 75 to 80 percent of their maximum heart rate—three times per week with a personal trainer lost nearly 12 pounds and gained just 1 pound after one year, compared to unsupervised and minimal-contact groups. If you're someone who struggles to stay accountable, hiring a personal trainer or downloading an app with regular check-ins can help, as can being a member of a supportive community. Feel your mojo starting to slide? Consider writing down your "why" as to why you want to lose weight and posting it somewhere you'll see it for inspiration on days you're less motivated. And get involved with in-person or on-line groups for support.

Secrets of People Who Lost Major Pounds—and Kept Them Off

Shedding triple digits (or nearly that) requires commitment, discipline and a lifestyle change that involves more than just food choices. Read inspiring stories of weight-loss success.

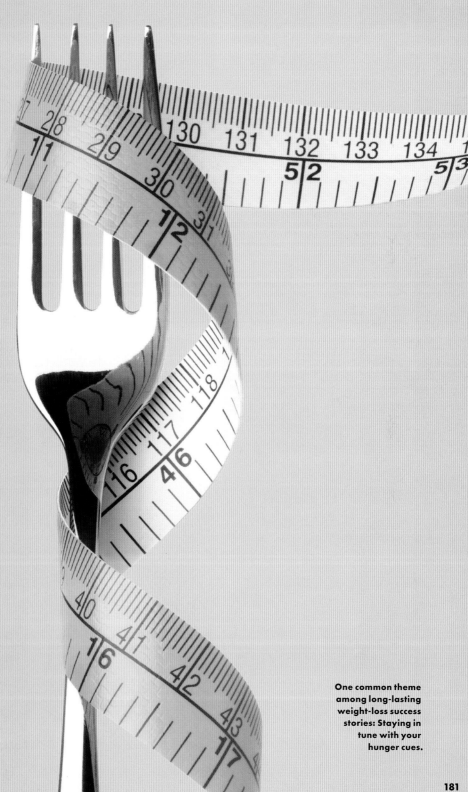

One common theme among long-lasting weight-loss success stories: Staying in tune with your hunger cues.

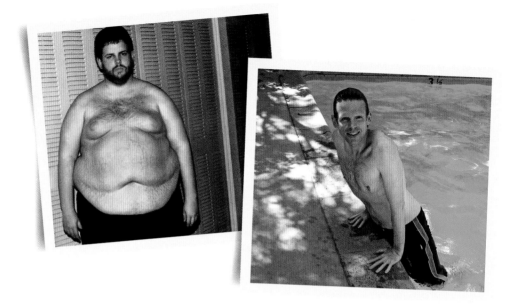

Gregg McBride

AGE 42
HEIGHT 5'11"
WEIGHT-LOSS STRATEGY
The DASH Diet and exercise
STARTING WEIGHT 450 lbs.
CURRENT WEIGHT 175 lbs.

I tried about every diet and every gimmick out there, usually more than once. I started gaining weight in first grade, which resulted in my parents putting me on a very strict diet. Although they were doing what they thought was right at the time (even under the advice of a doctor), this taught me "off (the diet)" and "on (the diet)" eating behaviors—which led to excessive fasting, dieting and bingeing. Any weight I lost would be eventually replaced with even more weight.

At the age of 27, I started trying to lose weight the old-fashioned way—through diet and exercise (mostly cardio: walking at first, and then graduating to aerobics classes). I gave up my daily diet-soda habit as well. I didn't restrict any food group, since restricting food always led to bingeing in the past. My goal was simple: to live a moderate and balanced life. I tried to eat as much "clean" or "fresh" food as possible—no additives, preservatives, artificial flavors or chemicals of any kind.

Breakfast would often be dry toast and fruit; lunch would usually be a salad (greens, tomatoes, a few other fresh vegetables) with a protein source (usually turkey), with balsamic vinegar mixed with a little Dijon mustard and pepper as a dressing. Dinner would usually be a protein source (chicken, fish) and a steamed vegetable (usually sprinkled with garlic and balsamic vinegar—no salt). If I had to snack, I'd eat fresh fruit. Initially, these foods tasted like cardboard to me, since I was so used to fast food and other junk foods that have lots of additives and unnecessary ingredients. Within a couple of weeks, my taste buds changed—and I found that a delicious Fuji apple could be as tasty to me as a bowl of ice cream.

Seeing the scale go down was exciting, but suddenly having to give up my 60-inch belt (which I'd been wearing out) was the most rewarding. I'll never forget the first time I could go into a store and pick out a pair of jeans (42 waist, the first time). It felt amazing! My new habits helped me lose 275 pounds in one year! I learned to combine all the tenets for weight loss—healthy food, exercise, good sleep and drinking water—to maintain it.

Steve Rosenthal

AGE 49
HEIGHT 5'8"
WEIGHT-LOSS STRATEGY
Keto and walking
STARTING WEIGHT 318 lbs.
CURRENT WEIGHT 228 lbs.

I created several smaller goals so that I could keep myself focused on the endgame. First, I wanted to get below 300 pounds. After that, 285, 275 and 250 were my goals. Recently, I had to buy a pair of size-34 pants—and I want to get to the size 32 I wore in high school. I stayed true to my initial promise to myself to not set new goals until I achieve the current ones and that's helped me stay focused and successful losing nearly 100 pounds eating keto.

I started off following The Keto Diet strictly but now that I'm closer to my goal weight after nearly a year, I slowly added more carbs into my diet (like fruits) but I'm still losing weight. I enjoy eating keto foods (like meat and eggs), but in the beginning, I had to get creative with ways to vary my proteins and fats. I've added avocados into my diet much more frequently and I find that I really enjoy them. I keep my meals interesting and fresh by following keto blogs and Facebook groups for recipes, as well as trying to take traditional recipes and make them keto.

What works for me is eating breakfast and lunch every day, and dinner about four days a week. On the other days, I skip dinner because I will have eaten a late lunch or I'm doing a modified intermittent fast. I walk for exercise at least five days a week, setting daily steps goals with a Fitbit monitor.

Some family members have decided to try keto after seeing my success and I've heard from real-life and online friends that my progress or recipes have spurred them to try something different, which is a great feeling. I fully intend to remain "keto-ish" as a lifetime goal.

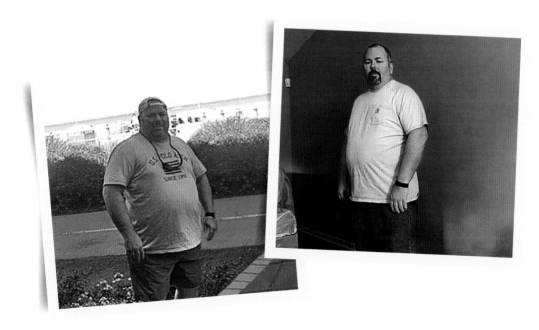

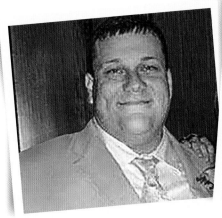
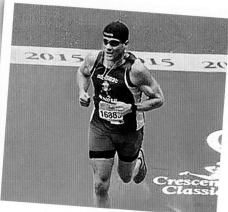

Josh LaJaunie

AGE 41
HEIGHT 6'3"
WEIGHT-LOSS STRATEGY Paleo and plant-based
STARTING WEIGHT 420 lbs.
CURRENT WEIGHT 190 lbs.

I was always going on diets and tried them all—Atkins, Weight Watchers, Jenny Craig, high-protein, high-fat, fasting, powders, shakes and pills—and they all worked great for a little while. I would lose 80, 90 even 100 pounds and reach whatever my latest magical target weight was. Then, to celebrate, I would go right back to the foods and beverages that had made me fat in the first place—and gain back every single pound plus some. I didn't have a clue about what a sustainable way of eating was, and I was completely ignorant of the science of nutrition, so I had no idea that certain diets simply cannot be maintained indefinitely, even if they are wicked effective at helping shed excess weight at first.

The plan I finally was able to sustain turned out to be one without gimmicks and without counting: Paleo. Basically, I looked for foods that our ancestors could have reliably sourced and made them the centerpiece of my plate—lots of unprocessed and minimally processed plant foods that are multicolored and low in calories. I used to love consuming huge volumes of food, so I needed to find foods that could fill me up without loading up on the calories. Greens, potatoes and sweet potatoes, vegetables, fruits, mushrooms and legumes were all foods that I lost weight eating, no matter how much I shoved in my mouth. And they still make up the lion's share of my diet today. I'm mostly a plant-based eater now. The multicolored part is more about health than weight loss, since the colors in plants signify different micronutrients, antioxidants, phytochemicals and other wonder molecules designed to keep us free from chronic inflammation and disease. By "eating the rainbow" of fruits and vegetables, I was following a simple rule that gave me all the nutrients my body needed in exactly the right amounts and ratios. And because I got healthier and healthier, the diet was much more sustainable than the others I'd tried.

Once I started losing weight, I began to realize that the journey and outcome was about far more than how many pounds I weighed. The dirty little secret of weight loss was that the minute I thought I'd achieved my goal, I was actually beginning my journey. Now that I'm living a life in harmony with nature and my highest self, I find joy in living, not in food. After a few years of progressing along the path of easy walks and slow jogs, I ultimately turned into a marathoner. I've competed in more than 10 marathons and have run longer-distance races: 50 miles; 50ks (at least six times); a 100k; and a 100-mile race. I now find joy in my physical capacity, going from being a guy who couldn't fit into a booth at a restaurant to someone who can do five sets of five pull-ups a day.

Meagan Kerans

AGE 33
HEIGHT 5'10"
WEIGHT-LOSS STRATEGY
Mediterranean and intuitive eating
STARTING WEIGHT 390 lbs.
CURRENT WEIGHT 286 lbs.

I've struggled with my weight my entire life. I was always a lot bigger than the other kids in elementary school. Being overweight became part of my identity. And when you are overweight, people offer lots of unsolicited advice, so I finally got to the point where I threw away every piece of advice I'd ever been given and started eating clean and listening to my body.

While I've tried many diets, the one thing that's made me most successful is cutting out processed foods. I started "shopping the perimeter" and eating mostly vegetables, fruits, whole grains, eggs, cheese, yogurt, fish and very little meat. I find that I feel best and see the best results when I eat high-protein, moderate-fat and moderate-carb. Most of the carbs I eat are from vegetables, like sweet potatoes, beets and squash. Food is pretty social. It's nice to know that I have the flexibility to have brunch with friends and keep my day on track by eating healthy foods I spot on the menu and keeping an eye on what I eat the rest of the day.

My relationship with my body has changed so much. I've come to a place where I'm genuinely thankful for it and everything it's capable of. After I started losing weight, I found the confidence to leave my longtime job and become a flight attendant, since I love to travel. I enjoy my job so much, and it's not lost on me that I'd never have been physically able to do it had I not lost the weight.

I enjoy being active and seeing the world like this. I love hiking when I travel, from mountains in Denver to a coastal trail in Greece. I was able to scuba dive on the Great Barrier Reef. I'm doing so many things I simply could not have done at almost 400 pounds. Losing the weight and learning how to fuel my body with healthy food changed my life.

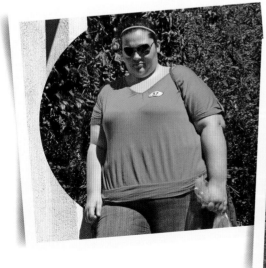

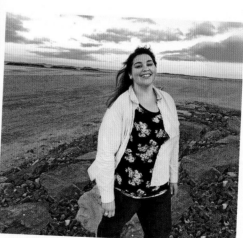

COVER Dirtydog_Creative/Getty Images **2-3** Prostock-Studio/Getty Images **4-5** From Left: wundervisuals/Getty Images. kasia2003/ Getty Images. Westend61/Getty Images. The Picture Pantry/Getty Images. kyoshino/Getty Images **6-7** Prostock-Studio/Getty Images **8-9** gilaxia/Getty Images **10-11** PeopleImages/Getty Images **12-13** PeopleImages/Getty Images. Jure Gasparic/EyeEm/Getty Images **14-15** From left: PeopleImages/Getty Images. kgfoto/Getty Images **16-17** PeopleImages/Getty Images **18-19** Westend61/Getty Images **20-21** Science Photo Library/Getty Images **22-23** From left: DNY59/Getty Images. ShotPrime/Getty Images **24-25** From left: Flashpop/Getty Images. Burazin/Getty Images **26-27** bhofack2/Getty Images **28-29** From left: IGphotography/Getty Images. amesy/ Getty Images **30-31** haoliang/Getty Images (2) **32-33** From left: Elena_Danileiko/Getty Images. courtesy Ocean's Halo **34-35** Influx Productions/Getty Images **36-37** SDI Productions/Getty Images **38-39** From left: amphotora/Getty Images. fcafotodigital/Getty Images. courtesy government **40-41** © Emoke Szabo/Getty Images **42-43** From left: OksanaKiian/Getty Images. xamtiw/Getty Images **44-45** From left: Samohin/Getty Images. istetiana/Getty Images **46-47** From left: YelenaYemchuk/Getty Images. naumoid/ Getty Images **48-49** Foodcollection RF/Getty Images **50-51** wragg/Getty Images **52-53** From left: Lew Robertson/Getty Images. Creativ Studio Heinemann/Getty Images **54-55** From left: fotogal/Getty Images. Stígur Már Karlsson /Heimsmyndir/Getty Images **56-57** From left: wundervisuals/Getty Images. romiri/Getty Images. flubydust/Getty Images **58-59** Brian Hagiwara/Getty Images **60-61** sveta_zarzamora/Getty Images **62-63** bit245/Getty Images **64-65** topotishka/Getty Images **66-67** From left: Magone/ Getty Images. Moyo Studio/Getty Images **68-69** Richard Drury/Getty Images **70-71** From left: Ng Sok Lian/EyeEm/Getty Images. Foodcollection RF/Getty Images. ithinksky/Getty Images. fcafotodigital/Getty Images **72-73** Jamie Grill/Getty Images **74-75** Clockwise from top left: Jon Lovette/Getty Images. Jon Lovette/Getty Images. broadcastertr/Getty Images. Rico K_dder EyeEm/Getty Images. JamieB/Getty Images. Xinzheng/Getty Images. StockFood/Getty Images (2). THEPALMER/Getty Images. Science Photo Library/Getty Images **76-77** Clockwise from top left: Martin Kreppel/EyeEm/Getty Images. Jon Lovette/Getty Images. tuk69tuk/Getty Images. nycshooter/Getty Images. ALEAIMAGE/Getty Images. Pongasn68/Getty Images. R.Tsubin/Getty Images. Adam Smigielski/Getty Images. George Mdivanian/EyeEm/Getty Images. macida/Getty Images. Wong Sze Fei/EyeEm/ Getty Images. Science Photo Library/Getty Images **78-79** Mike Kemp/Getty Images/Getty Images **80-81** photka/Getty Images **82-83** OlgaMiltsova/Getty Images **84-85** From left: Nattawut Lakjit/EyeEm/Getty Images. fcafotodigital/Getty Images **86-87** From left: Pjjaruwan/Shutterstock. iStock/Getty Images **88-89** From left: Gabriel Vergani/EyeEm/Getty Images. Claudia Totir/Getty Images **90-91** From left: Nattawut Lakjit/EyeEm/Getty Images. Elena_Danileiko/Getty Images **92-93** EyeEm/Getty Images **94-95** From left: EyeEm/Getty Images. Johner Images/Getty Images **96-97** From left: alle12/Getty Images. anyaivanova/Getty Images **98-99** From left: R.Tsubin /Getty Images. Arx0nt/Getty Images **100-101** From left: Suzifoo/Getty Images. The Picture Pantry/Getty Images **102-103** From Left: EvgeniiAnd/Getty Images. Lumina Images/Getty Images **104-105** From left: Lew Robertson/Getty Images. rez-art/Getty Images **106-107** luchezar/Getty Images **108-109** From left: kasia2003/Getty Images. baibaz/Getty Images **110-111** Claudia Totir/Getty Images **112-113** From left: Claudia Totir/Getty Images. LauriPatterson/Getty Images **114-115** From left: JakobFridholm/Getty images. Nungning20/Getty Images **116-117** Claudia Totir/Getty Images **118-119** Claudia Totir/Getty Images (2) **120-121** Claudia Totir/Getty Images **122-123** vaaseenaa/Getty Images **124-125** From left: eli_asenova/Getty Images. Claudia Totir/Getty Images **126-127** From left: Dimitris66/Getty Images. Dzevoniia/Getty Images **128-129** NoirChocolate/Getty Images **130-131** From left: kittimages/Getty Images. wmaster890/Getty Images **132-133** Martin Poole/Getty Images **134-135** Burcu Atalay Tankut/Getty Images **136-137** Claudia Totir/Getty Images **138-139** LauriPatterson/Getty Images **140-141** David Malan/Getty Images **142-143** From left: kyoshino/Getty Images. jenifoto/Getty Images **144-145** From left: Andrzej Siwiec / EyeEm/Getty Images. twomeows/Getty Images **146-147** nata_vkusidey/Getty Images **148-149** From left: los_angela/Getty Images. freeskyline/Getty Images **150-151** Kevin Kozicki/Getty Images **152-153** Leonardo Patrizi/Getty Images **154-155** Leonardo Patrizi/Getty Images **156-157** From left: Leonardo Patrizi/Getty Images. PhotoAlto/Jana Hernette/Getty Images **158-159** Leonardo Patrizi/Getty Images **160-161** PeopleImages/Getty Images **162-163** JGI/Jamie Grill/Getty Images **164-165** From left: mammuth/Getty Images. Fototocam/Getty Images **166-167** From left: the_burtons/Getty Images. Peter Stark/Getty Images **168-169** skynesher/Getty Images **170-171** Westend61/Getty Images **172**: Clockwise from top left: Natalia Ganelin/Getty Images. Saturn_3/Getty Images. liangpv/ Getty Images. Steve Wisbauer/Getty Images. Anthony Harvie/Getty Images. DNY59/Getty Images. Natalia Ganelin/Getty Images. Susanne Kürth/EyeEm/Getty Images. sbayram/Getty Images. StockFood/Getty Images Floortje/Getty Images (2). Tony Cordoza/ Getty Images. Foodcollection RF/Getty Images. Sarah Saratonina/EyeEm/Getty Images. The Picture Pantry/Getty Images **173**: Floortje/Getty Images **174-175** LeoPatrizi/Getty Images **176-177** Jacobs Stock Photography Ltd/Getty Images **178-179** From left: Ivanko_Brnjakovic/Getty Images. luxcreative/Getty Images **180-181** Science Photo Library/Getty Images **182-183** Courtesy Subjects **184-185** Courtesy Subjects. photohampster/Getty Images. malerapaso/Getty Images **SPINE** mgkaya/Getty Images **BACK COVER** From top: anyaivanova/Getty Images. Kevin Kozicki/Getty Images. Claudia Totir/Getty Images

SPECIAL THANKS TO CONTRIBUTING WRITERS

Julie D. Andrews

Liz Josefsberg

Judy Koutsky

Nicole Kwan

Vanessa Voltolina Labue

SJ McShane

Lauren Mazzo

Katherine Schreiber

Celia Shatzman

Jenn Sinrich

Brittany Smith

Colleen Travers

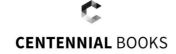

CENTENNIAL BOOKS

An Imprint of
Centennial Media, LLC
40 Worth St., 10th Floor
New York, NY 10013, U.S.A.

ISBN 978-1-951274-37-5

Distributed by
Simon & Schuster, Inc.
1230 Avenue of the Americas
New York, NY 10020, U.S.A.

For information about custom editions, special sales and premium and corporate purchases,
please contact Centennial Media at contact@centennialmedia.com.

Manufactured in China